FUELLED

TRANSFORM YOUR BODY
ENHANCE YOUR ENERGY
SUPERCHARGE YOUR LIFE

AGATHE REGINA HOLOWATINC, MLIS, INHC

Food photography by Nhuri Bashir
Foreword by Dr. Reid Robinson

Praise for Agathe Regina Holowatinc's
FUELLED

Wow!!! Definitely a must read for anyone who is ready to take control of their health and get FUELLED. Easy to follow delicious whole food recipes for the entire family. Everything looks so beautiful. Broccoli has never tasted so good! I just want Agathe to be my personal chef.

>-Teresa Perozzi, *Former WBA Middleweight world boxing champion, three time fittest in Bermuda female Crossfit competitor, wife, mom and owner of Body in Balance in Bermuda.*

FUELLED is essential reading for anyone looking to optimize their wellness, shed excess weight and increase their energy levels! The book is inspiring and insightful, and many "Ah-ha" moments await. Written in a practical and approachable way, the simplicity of the instructions are great, and cutting-edge topics like epigentics and phytonutrients are covered. As a clinical psychologist, I deeply admire Agathe's approach to the behavioural aspects involved in making a decision to change your life and to start on a new path towards healthy, life-giving and nourishing eating. Lifestyle factors such as sleep are also highlighted, which is very important. I believe that you need to look at your whole life if you want the best results. The FUELLED Real-Food Recipe Guide is fun and easy to follow and the photos are great! But mostly, I love that it places a heavy emphasis on plant-based foods as that is the way to go for your body, mind and spirit. I made a decision years ago to adopt a vegan lifestyle, and I feel very strongly about the amazing health benefits of eating plant-based – which include improved digestion, increased energy, better sleep, healthier weight, clearer skin, lower rates of chronic diseases, increased life expectancy, significant improvements in general health, performance, vitality, clarity and mental health...the list goes on! And not to mention the numerous environmental and ethical reasons to go plant-based...plus it just tastes so good! And, as the book states: "what is more convincing than *pleasure*?" Agathe Holowatinc is a passionate advocate of optimal well-being via education, inspiration, motivation and transformation and in her heart she wishes to help people live their lives to the fullest. FUELLED contains a powerful message of hope, transformation and creating an extraordinary life. I highly recommend this book!

> - Dr. Joti Samra, R.Psych., *Clinical Psychologist. Organizational, Research & Media Consultant. Host of Oprah Winfrey Network's Million Dollar Neighbourhood. Psychological Consultant to The Bachelor Canada. Provincially qualified BCABBA fitness competitor.* www.DrJotiSamra.com

---

If you want to make a change for the better this year, especially with your physical body, FUELLED is the book for you. It will educate and inspire you... and then show you how to really take action using the Real Food How-To Recipe Guide. It's easy to follow and everything looks incredibly delicious.

> - Jeffrey Baron, J.P., M.P., *Dad, Advisor and Former Minister of National Security (Bermuda).*

FUELLED offers us a fresh vision of optimal health achieved through nature's most fundamental gift – food. Agathe Holowatinc has created an easy blueprint for you to begin to transform your life from the inside out. Reading FUELLED is like having a conversation with your best friend about how you can begin to feel great in your own skin for no other reason than because you are worth it! Agathe writes with knowledge and clarity about cutting edge topics such as epigenetics and its relevance to your food and lifestyle choices in such an accessible way that you feel not only educated, but empowered to make changes in your life that will maximize your body's energy and vitality. FUELLED is a journey back to a simpler, wiser way of being in the world and relating to our food as the primary source of a healthy body, mind and spirit. As a yoga teacher, the foods I eat and the choices I make are guided by the ancient yogic principle of "sattva," or foods and behaviours which are light, pure and non-toxic to the body and the planet. The guidance that Agathe provides in FUELLED resonates deeply with this ancient yogic wisdom also. More than just a cookbook, it is an invitation to take control of your health and step into your personal power by starting where you are, and harnessing the power of the body to heal, rejuvenate and thrive when given the right FUEL!

    - Shanell Vaughn, M.A., E-RYT 200. *Yoga Teacher, Holistic Health Practitioner, Owner of Shambhala Bermuda.*

I have been looking for additional information to add to our wellness program for addicts in recovery. I have found it in FUELLED by Agathe Holowatinc. Recovery from drug addiction requires a multi-faceted approach and a reorientation on how to engage in self care. FUELLED helps us educate our clients on natural detoxification, and how proper nutrition can help the body and mind heal from years of abuse.

    - Dr Ernest Peets Jr., CFT, ICADC, *Clinical Manager of Turning Point Substance Abuse Program, Certified Family Therapist and Internationally Certified Addictions Counselor.*

FUELLED

TRANSFORM YOUR BODY
ENHANCE YOUR ENERGY
SUPERCHARGE YOUR LIFE

Agathe Regina Holowatinc, MLIS, INHC
Food photography by Nhuri Bashir
Foreword by Dr. Reid Robinson

FUEL = Food Unleashing Energy for Life™

FUELLED: Transform Your Body | Enhance Your Energy | Supercharge Your Life

Copyright © 2018 by Agathe Regina Holowatinc, MLIS, INHC

All rights reserved.

First Edition: February 2018

No part of this publication may be reproduced, distributed, or transmitted in any form or by any means, including photocopying, recording, or other electronic or mechanical methods, without the prior written permission of the author, except in the case of brief quotations embodied in critical reviews and certain other non-commercial uses permitted by copyright law. For permission requests, email info@fuelledlife.com.

This book contains advice and information relating to health care. It should be used to supplement rather than replace the advice of your doctor or another trained health professional. The advice and strategies contained in this book may not be suitable for all readers. Please speak to your healthcare provider if you have any questions about your own medical situation. All efforts have been made to assure the accuracy of the information contained in this book as of the date of publication. The publisher, author, IIN® and its employees, disclaim liability for any medical outcomes that may occur as a result of applying the methods suggested in this book.

For information contact:
Agathe Regina Holowatinc
http://fuelledlife.com

Food Photography by Nhuri Bashir
http://nhuribashir.com/

Book interior design by Jana Rade of Impact Studios
http://www.impactstudiosonline.com/

ISBN: 978-0-947481-16-2 (hardcover edition)
ISBN: 978-0-947481-14-8 (paperback edition)
ISBN: 978-0-947481-15-5 (eBook edition)

Printed and bound in the United States of America

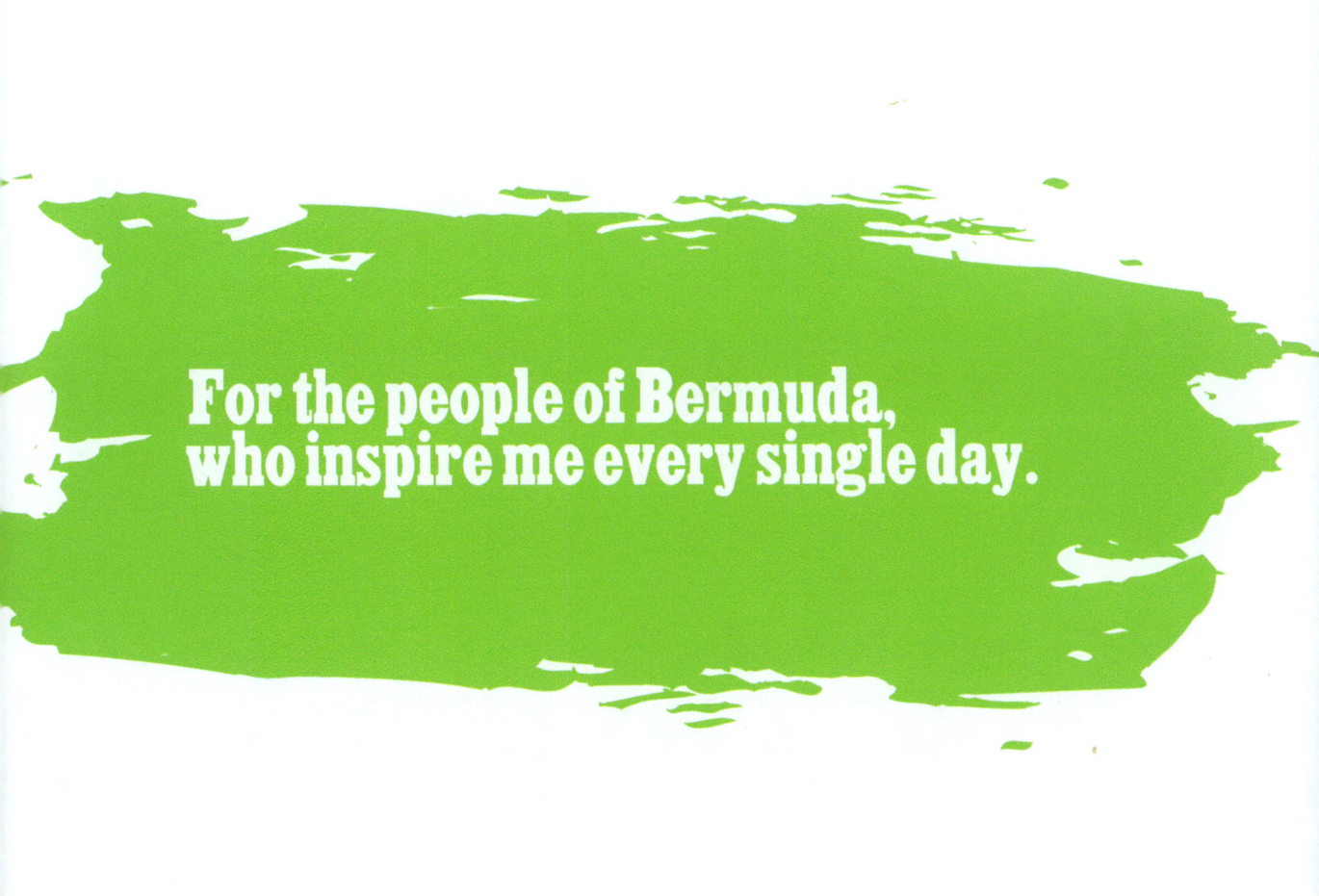

FOOD
FUEL
Unleashing
Energy for
LIFE™

CONTENTS

FOREWORD.................................XV

INTRODUCTION 13

PART 1: EDUCATE—........................ 21
Raise the Bar on What Food Can Do For You

PART 2: INSPIRE—......................... 77
Fight Your Fears, Find Your Fire & Visualize Your Best Self

PART 3: TRANSFORM—..................... 89
FUELLED Real Food How-To Recipe Guide

A FINAL NOTE 245

PART 4: REFERENCES 247

FOREWORD

Modern chronic diseases, also known as "diseases of civilization," which include, but are not limited to, cancer, heart disease and diobesity, cause around 70% of all deaths in the Western world. Chronic illness rates are rising exponentially worldwide in all age groups. Type 2 diabetes, once known as adult-onset diabetes, is now pandemic in children and adolescents, who are being prescribed cholesterol and anti-hypertensive medication, and, for the first time in two centuries, are expected to have a shorter lifespan than their parents. That's right: it has been reported that the current generation of children in America could have a life expectancy shorter than their parents if childhood obesity is left unchecked. And they risk spending their later years in very poor health. The reality is that the obesity pandemic has diminished quality of life, overwhelmed health systems and bankrupt families around the globe.

And yet, chronic diseases are largely preventable diseases. There has been absolutely no change in the human genome during the current period of exponential increase in chronic illness rates, prescription rates, and spending on pharmaceutical drugs. These diseases, once thought to be due to genetic predetermination, have now been shown to be the direct result of lifestyle choices. The lifestyle choices we make each day have a greater impact on our health and vitality than anything else. Diet has been known for many years to play a key role as a risk factor for chronic diseases, and so, in turn, it plays a key a role in the prevention of these same chronic diseases. What this means is that we have a choice and power over our longevity and the quality of our lives.

There is nothing magical about human physiology that allows us to eat toxic or deficient diets without severe health consequences. Humans are possibly the world's sickest animal species. Why? Because the prevailing belief system is that we get sick from bad luck, bad germs, bad genes, old age and bad weather. That's just bad science.

Are you ready to shift your mindset? FUELLED is a succinct, eloquent, evidence-based presentation that inspires the genetic program deep inside of us to thrive. Holowatinc writes from a position supported by a wave of change in the scientific community. In the following pages she underscores how, from a genetic perspective, human physiology has changed very little in the past 40,000 years, yet our Standard American Diet (SAD) has made a massive turn for the worst. To elicit fundamental change, Holowatinc uses education and inspiration to help you achieve what you are genetically programmed for: health and vitality.

As a wellness practitioner, researcher and educator, FUELLED inspires me to make those last tweaks in my diet, which are made easy with these simple, colourful and delicious recipes. If you are looking for change because you are "tired of being sick and tired," curious about "the hype," interested in getting lean without deprivation, or you just know that there's more out there for you – this book is for you. If you are truly ready to see what becoming healthy and living your most vibrant, amazing, driven and energized life could feel like...this book will get you well on your way. Don't expect to feel hungry after eating these nutrient-dense meals. Expect MORE productive energy, more balanced moods, less bloating, less suffering, and less brain fog, just to name a few benefits.

Get ready to be "FUELLED" for life.

- Dr. Reid G. Robinson, D.C., Chiropractor, Wellness Practitioner, Owner and Founder of Inside Out Wellness Centre.

FUELLED

INTRO

> "The future depends on what we do in the present."
>
> —Mahatma Gandhi

If you are like most people, I imagine there are specific goals you have for your health and your life.

Perhaps you want to dramatically increase the energy you have on a daily basis, beat fatigue, shed unnecessary and unwanted weight, be proud of the physical state of your body, and, of course, look younger and feel sexier. Perhaps you are tired of being *sick* and *tired* and feeling held back in life. Maybe you want to detoxify and cleanse your body, sharpen your thinking, and stop the poisoning you feel you might have been doing to yourself. Or perhaps you just know that there's more out there for you and you are truly ready to see what the road to becoming healthy and living your most vibrant, amazing, driven and energized life could feel like.

Does any of this sound familiar?

If so, this book could very well be a turning point in your life.

This book is about changing your health destiny. It's about making choices that are right for your health instead of relying on chance, luck, 'good' genes or 'bad' genes to determine your weight, energy levels or health outcomes. It's about taking your life and your health into your own hands, and changing the course of the future for the better, no matter where you are right now. This book is here to educate you, inspire you, motivate you and then show you exactly how to make the changes you need to make to get from where you are to where you want to be. It is about showing you how to feed your body with the **FUEL** it needs for sustained weight loss, *optimal* health and enhanced energy for the long term. Because you have the power to do it, starting right now, starting TODAY. Don't wait until you are sick, or sicker. "The future depends on what we do in the present," Mahatma Gandhi so wisely instructed us.

I believe that energy, good health and vitality are the keys to living a magnificent life and that is the basis of the FUELLED philosophy. I wrote this book so that I could help you unlock the secret of true **FUEL** in your life, where **FUEL** is an acronym for *Food Unleashing Energy for Life.* This acronym is the guiding principle for this book and the life changing journey you are just about to embark on.

FUELLED is the roadmap for the next stage in your health journey and the key to gaining your nutritional advantage in life. It will help you navigate through the jungle of confusing and conflicting diet and nutrition information out there and present to you the fundamentals of a new and revolutionary way of viewing food and your body. Once you decide to start on the path of healthy, life-giving and nutrient-dense eating, FUELLED will help you bridge the gap between where you are and where you want to be. And it's not going to be complicated – the key to getting FUELLED is to take in maximum nourishment from amazing foods and fluids the majority of the time so that your cells are flourishing and you are living a vibrant life. Reading this book is the first step in becoming more energized and feeling revitalized and rejuvenated on a daily basis.

You see, my mission is to help you gain your energy edge, shed unwanted weight and close the gap between where you are now and where you want to be through FUELLING your body so it works at an optimal level - helping you achieve a vibrant and fulfilling life you might have thought previously unimaginable for yourself so that I can see you succeed in the progressive realization of worthy goals and dreams after that. Because achieving optimal health is *the best* springboard for achieving all of your biggest dreams.

Herophilus, an ancient Greek physician born in 335 BC, said: "When health is absent, wisdom cannot reveal itself, art cannot manifest, strength cannot fight, wealth becomes useless, and intelligence cannot be applied."

You have the power to change your health and your body. And you simply cannot experience an *extraordinary* quality of life without the vehicle that's going to help you create it. Once you adopt the practices in this book and get FUELLED, you'll emerge a true warrior — ready to power through anything because you are unstoppable!

The choice is yours. Get FUELLED today for a healthier and happier, more powerful and promising tomorrow.

I wish you all the success in the world as you embark on this journey of achieving optimal health and creating an abundant, passionate and **FUELLED** life!

YOU'VE GOT THIS.

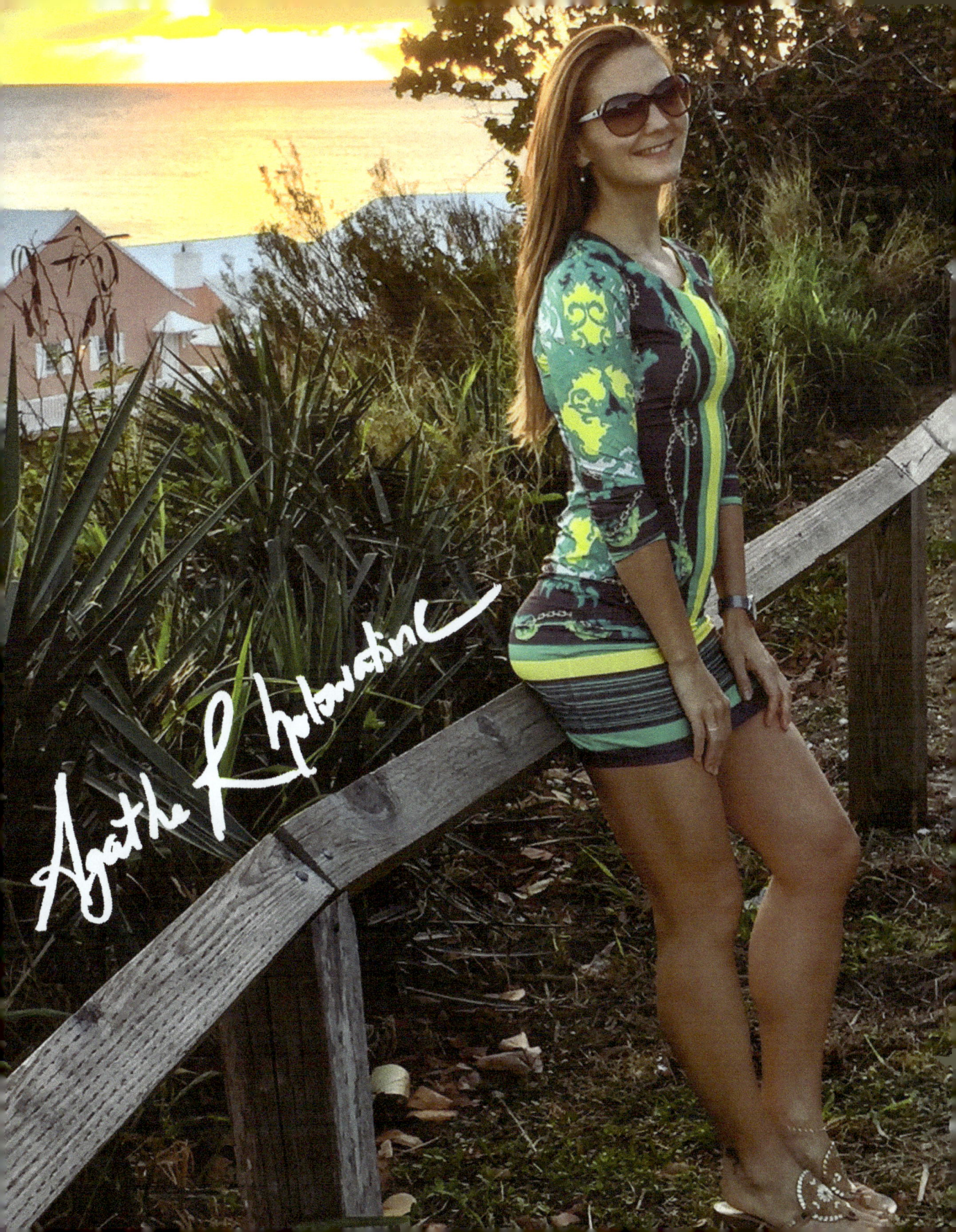

How to Use This Book

What makes this book different is that it is divided into 3 meaningful sections that represent the steps it takes for you to progress on your journey to getting **FUELLED** successfully: Educate > Inspire > Transform. Written as part education, part inspiration and part Real Food Recipe Guide, it is a comprehensive, easy-to-read handbook chock-full of simple recipes, instructions and inspirational messages to help you progress in your journey towards achieving better cellular health through optimal, nutrient-dense eating.

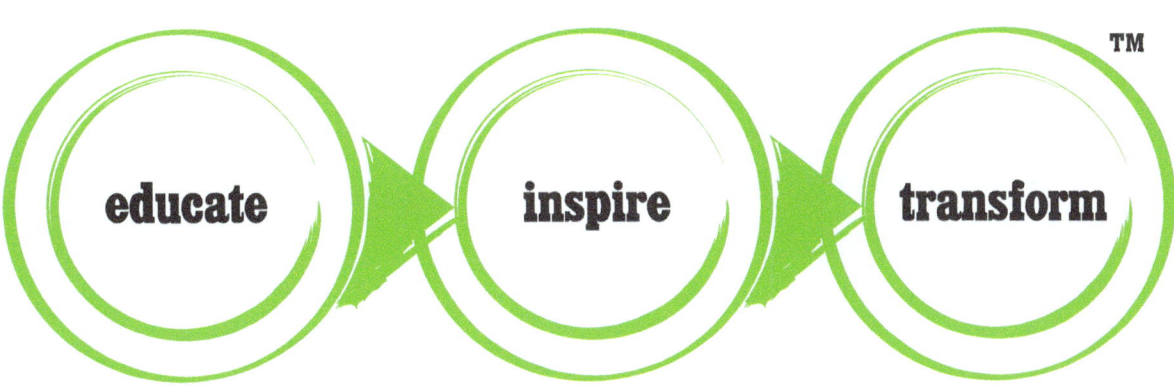

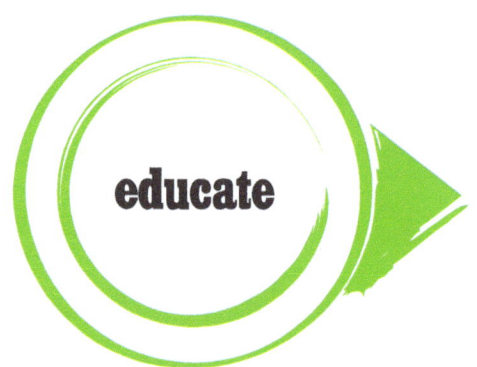

The first step to becoming your best self is found in *Educate*. You have some stuff to learn, or to unlearn in some cases. The truth is that most of us didn't learn about eating good food in school or at least not in a way that really stuck and made an impact on our attitude, behavior and wellbeing over the long term. Our parents, caretakers and communities might not have passed down the best beliefs or practices surrounding food and how to eat well. In this section, we examine your current beliefs surrounding health, your body and eating. Then I challenge you to consider whether your beliefs are serving you, are in your best interests, or whether it's time for an overhaul of your health and wellness mindset. I encourage you to adopt a better philosophy towards health, energy and how to FUEL your body at the cellular level.

But before embarking on a total overhaul of your health and wellness mindset, it's important to first *Educate* yourself about nutrition, how food impacts the cells, and your body's vital needs. This section provides all the information you need to know about which foods, nutrients and supplements FUEL the body for maximum health benefits.

I will introduce you to the transformative power of nutritional energy in creating and sustaining a level of optimal health, energy and vitality you might have thought previously unimaginable for yourself. This is all based on the core principle of simply selecting, preparing and eating *real* food. No diets, no gimmicks – just biology. By the time you've finished this section, you will have the knowledge to understand how *real* food provides the best FUEL for life, and, consequently, you will have the knowledge to understand how to unlock the potential of **FUEL = Food Unleashing Energy for Life**.

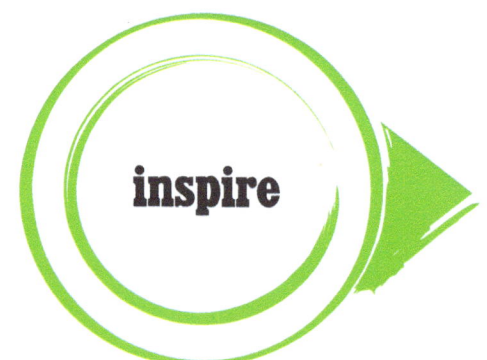

In between education and transformation comes inspiration. Without the proper vision and motivation, our chances of successfully achieving our goals and realizing our passions are greatly diminished. In other words, information alone is rarely what motivates people to uplevel (that is, to improve or enhance) their health and their lifestyle. It's necessary that we feel *inspired* to make different choices, adopt better eating habits and envision a new future for ourselves. This is a key ingredient that's missing from most diets and nutrition fads. This section will help you uncover your "Why" — that is, help you establish the motivation behind "why" you're pursuing becoming a more vibrant and healthy You. You are far more likely to reach any goal that you have set for yourself when you can clearly articulate your reasons for wanting to achieve it. Following that, I will support you as you tap into the awesome power of visualization to create a vision of success as relates to you living a healthy, happy and energized life. In summary, *Inspire* lifts your heart and your spirit towards eating healthier today and encourages you to really take that very important first step. Because whether or not you feel inspired directly impacts your day-to-day decision making, eating choices and your potential for successfully upleveling your nutrition game and achieving optimal health in the short and long term.

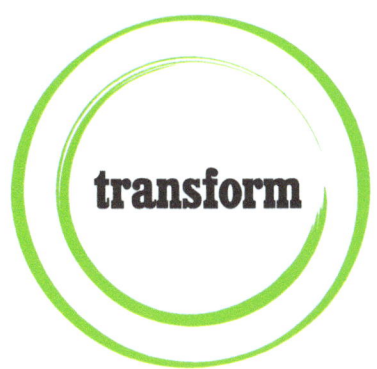

It's time to apply all of the knowledge contained in the *Educate* section of this book and all of the passion gained from the *Inspire* section of this book to FUEL your cells and propel yourself forward. It's time to transform your life and alter your reality. The *Transform* section of this book shows you how to apply your knowledge and create remarkable, easy and delicious meals that form the backbone of a healthier, more vibrant you. I don't blame you for wanting to jump straight into it.

In other words, this section shows you *how* to transform your life, starting with the basics and a simple, FUELLED Real Food How-To Recipe Guide. There are over 100 delicious and easy recipes that will enable you to FUEL your body in the best way — and get FUELLED for the next phase of your life!

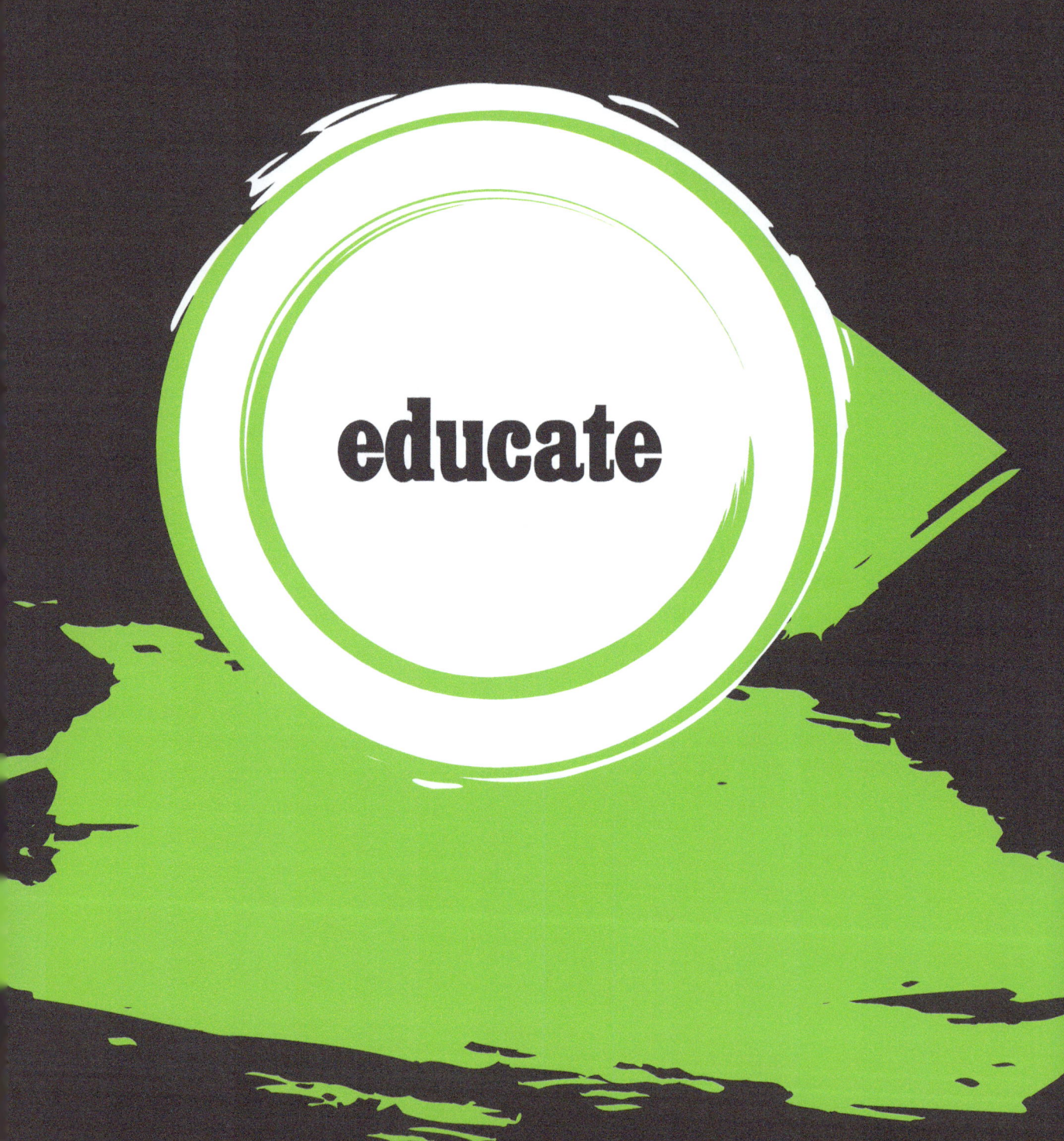

Knowledge Is Power.

What you are about to read has the potential to dramatically improve your life.

Have you ever wondered why there are a seemingly endless number of diets and healthy eating trends? Yeah, me too. All of those diets can be confusing and overwhelming. Worse, some may even be misleading and downright unhealthy, preying on our personal anxieties and self-consciousness.

It's time for a total overhaul of your health and wellness mindset. It's time to finally learn how food can nourish your cells. How *real* food has the power to harness the best from your cells. How *real* food has the power to activate an enormous amount of untapped potential within you. It's time to learn how to create and sustain a level of optimal health, energy and vitality that you previously thought unimaginable by educating yourself on how *real* food provides the **FUEL** for life.

It's time to radically transform the way you view the food on your plate and the liquid in your cup.

This section will educate you on exactly why you need to *Raise the Bar* on what you expect food can do for you. Because it can do a hell of a lot and you need to know about it.

And remember, as author Jordan Phoenix writes, "When we educate ourselves, we learn new things that we were previously unaware of. This gives us the ability to make better decisions, come up with more evolved and intelligent thoughts, improve the lives of ourselves and those around us, and thus makes us more valuable people overall (2017)."

The Power of the Human Body and our Genes

"You have been given a nearly flawless gift that has been in the making for over two million years. It has been refined and polished over countless generations to provide you with optimal health, functionality and longevity."

– David Perlmutter, M.D.

In the past, we thought of genes as unchangeable. That is, we thought that the genes inside our cells today were exactly the same as the genes we were born with. That they were set and fixed. And if you had parents who carried the genes for cancer, diabetes, Alzheimer's or just that good ol' "fat gene" then you were destined to suffer from that same ailment. Or, on the other hand, if you had great genes from your parents, you just automatically looked younger and were more handsome or beautiful and healthier than everyone else. For decades, the prevailing wisdom was that, in many ways, our biology determined our destiny. However, new research is challenging this theory. "It's time to explode such rigid notions," write Deepak Chopra and Rudolph E. Tanzi in *Super Genes: Unlock the Astonishing Power of Your DNA for Optimum Health and Well-Being* (p. 1, 2015).

EPIGENETICS

Today, scientists are becoming very interested in the emerging science of epigenetics, which means "above" or "on top of" genetics. In fact, it is one of the fastest-growing areas of science and something you need to know more about. I'll provide only a very brief and high level description of it here. Where *genetics* looks at our DNA, our genetic code, *epigenetics* looks at mechanisms other than those within the DNA sequence that will affect the activity of a gene and override some of the principles of genetics. Because all of the cells in our body contain an identical genetic code, epigenetic mechanisms control whether certain areas of the genome can be accessed or not and which of your genes may be expressed – for better or for worse. Biologist Nessa Carey states that "When scientists talk about epigenetics they are referring to all the cases in which the genetic code alone isn't enough to describe what's happening—there must be something else going on as well"(p.6, 2012). So, stay with me here, epigenetics refers to external modifications to DNA, typically identified as the addition or removal of small chemical groups at specific regions of the DNA, that do not change the underlying genetic code but that still play a significant role in regulating the specific expression of genes. Basically, these "external modifications" are chemical reactions brought on by processes outside of your DNA, including processes that are brought on by the consumption of specific nutrients and bioactive components from the foods you eat and the liquids you drink, that have been found to activate or deactivate parts of your genome that will either create better or worse health outcomes for you. That is because these changes in gene expression alter the functions of cells, and the very nature of the cells themselves. Epigenetics is revolutionary in that it reveals that both the environment and our individual lifestyle can directly interact with the genome to influence notable epigenetic changes. In the Foreword to the book *Effortless Healing, 9 Simple Ways to Sidestep Illness, Shed Excess Weight, and Help Your Body Fix Itself* (2016), written by Dr. Joseph Mercola, Dr. David Perlmutter states: "As it turns out, the notion that our DNA represents a fixed and immutable code is now looked upon as antiquated science. What we've come to understand is that our genetic code is actually aggressively dynamic in its expression" (2015). In other words, and in terms of achieving optimal health, we are seeing more and more how the behavior of your genes can be modified and impacted by external interventions, such as nutritional interventions, to improve health outcomes, by altering the function and nature of our cells. In a very real way, epigenetics has revolutionized our understanding of the structure and behaviour of all biological life. Your genes and health destiny are not concrete and set in stone from the day you are conceived. There is much more to it than that, especially when it comes to disease prevention and achieving optimal health.

Super Genes

The book *Super Genes: Unlock the Astonishing Power of Your DNA for Optimum Health and Well-Being* (2015), a New York Times bestseller written by Deepak Chopra, M.D. and Rudolph E. Tanzi, PhD. (the Joseph P. and Rose F. Kennedy Professor of Neurology at Harvard University, and Director of the Genetics and Aging Research Unit at Massachusetts General Hospital), dives into the science of epigenetics and then brings it home, explaining how the theory applies to our day-to-day life, health and wellbeing. Even though they admit that the science is still in its infancy, they argue that epigenetics shows us that our genes are *dynamic*, responding to physical, emotional, and possibly even mental changes in our body, mind and lifestyle (p. 1, 2015). Because genes are now understood to be controlled by external signals outside of our cells, according to Chopra and Tanzi, the foods we eat, our lifestyle, our gut bacteria and even our thoughts and perception of events can have an impact our genes, and influence how they respond – for better or for worse.

"Your genes are fluid, dynamic and responsive to everything you think and do," write Chopra and Tanzi in *Super Genes*. "The news everyone should hear is that gene activity is largely under our control. That's the breakthrough idea emerging from the new genetics" (p. 1, 2015).

The idea that the genes you inherited are the predictor of your future health is outdated. It's time to embrace the understanding that you have the power to make choices that optimize how your genes behave.

And further to the point, Chopra and Tanzi state that:

"The new genetics can be simplified in a single phrase: we are learning how to make our genes help us. Instead of allowing your bad genes to hurt you and your good genes to give you a break in life, which used to be the prevailing view, you should think of the super genome as a willing servant who can help you direct the life you want to live." (p. 4, 2015)

NUTRITION AND EPIGENETICS

> "In the nutritional field, epigenetics is exceptionally important, because nutrients and bioactive food components can modify epigenetic phenomena and alter the expression of genes at the transcriptional level."
>
> - Choi and Friso in *Epigentics: A New Bridge Between Nutrition and Health* (2010)

Right now, epigenetics research is flourishing in new fields, with studies that focus on inflammation, obesity, insulin resistance, type 2 diabetes, immune disease, cardiovascular diseases and neurodegenerative diseases. These studies are providing us with exciting insight into how we can use nutrients and bioactive food components for maintaining our health and preventing diseases through *modifiable epigenetic mechanisms*. Basically, they are showing us how nutrients can reverse or change certain epigenetic phenomena, thereby modifying the expression of genes critical to cellular processes and observable characteristics of an individual (or animal). Epigenetic research studies had traditionally had traditionally focused on aging-associated processes, the formation of cancers and the prevention of pediatric developmental diseases (early life development), but today they're expanding out to include studies that can help us understand how our diets can help us or hurt us, and, more specifically, how essential nutrients can help us mobilize our *epigenetic* nutritional advantage.

Here is a very brief glimpse into what we now know to be true about how food can have an epigenetic influence on our health and well-being:

- A well known study published in 2008 showed that honeybees grow to be either fertile queen bees or sterile worker bees depending on whether they were fed royal jelly or beebread, even though the larvae are genetically identical (Kucharski *et al.*, 2008).
- Your mother's diet during pregnancy can affect your epigenome in ways that stick with you into adulthood. In another well known and often cited study, referred to as "The Dutch Famine Study," researchers examined whether gestational exposure to famine (malnutrition), in this case, the one that occurred during the *Hongerwinter* in Holland in 1944 (during World War II), could be associated with chronic diseases in adulthood. As expected, babies born during the famine often had severe health issues. Those in the womb in the 3rd to 9th months of pregnancy during the famine were born underweight, however, those

babies in the 1st trimester near the end of the famine, just as food supplies were returning, were born larger than average. Furthermore, adults born during the famine were highly prone to obesity compared to adults born outside the famine (Lumey *et al.,* 2006; Chopra and Tanzi, 2015; Carey, 2012).

- Studies in Agouti mice have also shown that when a pregnant mother's diet has too little folate or choline before or just after birth, it causes certain regions of the genome of her offspring to be impacted for life, resulting in offspring that are prone to diabetes, cancer, cardiovascular disease and obesity. Also, typically her offspring have a yellow coat and are obese, but if the pregnant mother's diet was supplemented with folic acid, choline, vitamin B12 and betaine, her offspring had a brown coat (a profound change in phenotype), were slim and healthy. This study showed that dietary exposures can have long-term consequences for looks, growth and health (Dolinoy *et al.,* 2006).
- Eating sweet, fatty foods during pregnancy has been linked to Attention-Deficit Hyperactivity Disorder (ADHD) in children (Rijlaarsdam, J. *et al.,*2016).
- B vitamins have been shown to protect against harmful epigenetic effects of air pollution (Zhong, J. *et al.,* 2017).
- Curcumin, commonly known as turmeric, is one of the most powerful and promising chemopreventive and anticancer agents, and epidemiological evidence demonstrates that people who incorporate high doses of this spice in their diets have a lower incidence of cancer (Wargovich, 1997; Wilken *et al.,* 2011; Reuter *et al.,* 2011; Boyanapalli *et al.,* 2015).
- A 2016 study published in the *Proceedings of the National Academy of Sciences*, has found that Vitamins A and C aren't just good for your health, they affect your DNA too. In this study, researchers uncovered that these vitamins help erase epigenetic marks from the genome, meaning that they help them to regress from their current state into a more embryonic state. This has incredible implications for regenerative medicine because if you are able to return a cell back to its original state then you might be able to reprogram it into another cell (i.e. brain cells to heart cells). This shows us that epigenetics is reversible. We have been able to reverse some of the bad states, while keeping the good, using vitamins C and A (Hore *et al.*).

These are only a few examples of the increasing number of studies that depict how epigenetic variation can be modified by nutritional interventions to improve, or, in the case of the famine, to worsen, health outcomes (Burdge *et al.,* 2012).

IMPLICATIONS

In the forward to the book *Effortless Healing, 9 Simple Ways to Sidestep Illness, Shed Excess Weight, and Help Your Body Fix Itself* (2015), David Perlmutter, MD, states: "The profound upside of this new paradigm is that it reveals that each of us has the opportunity to modify our own genetic expression and change our health destiny."

Clearly, what we are learning from the emerging field of epigenetics has huge implications on how we can ultimately improve the quality of our lives, our energy levels and our health outcomes. The mindset that comes from this field really enables us to see how *we* have the power to immediately start to transform the quality of our lives today. We possess this gift of the human body and all the power it holds. And our lifestyle is where the transformation starts to take place. Where, by making simple, better choices, we can activate the potential our genes hold for optimal health, vitality, wellbeing and for enhancing the quality of our lives. "They've become our strongest allies for personal renewal," Chopra and Tanzi affirm (2015). The foods we eat, the fluids we drink, the environments we spend time in, the amount of exercise we get, the people we hang out with, the activities we take part in, the beliefs we hold and our perception of ourselves, our lives and our circumstances – all things outside of our cells – affect our genetic code at a cellular level. They affect how our genes respond – for better or for worse – and, therefore, they direct our health outcomes. Therefore, we can do things to positively influence the expression of our genes to improve and maintain our health over the long term. And, if you're concerned about all the damage you might have already done through your food and lifestyle choices to-date, you can breathe a slight sigh of relief, as some studies, like I mentioned above with vitamins A and C, show that, yes, epigenetic modifications are reversible. It is even said that your genes respond to what you do moment to moment – so every moment presents you with a new chance for a healthier and happier tomorrow.

There it is folks. That's the scoop you need to know. That's the revolutionary new idea that the concept of **FUEL[LED]** – *Food Unleashing Energy for Life* – stands on. You have the power to make choices that optimize how your genes behave, especially when it comes to nutrition. The emerging science of epigenetics reveals that your body can be changed as you uplevel your thinking, eating, lifestyle and environment. With a mindset like this, you can reach for a state of health and fulfillment that you might never have thought possible before. What can be more fascinating?

The emerging science of epigenetics suggests that your short and long-term health can be determined by none other than you. And in this book you will learn how FUELLING your body can alter your health for many decades to come, regardless of the genes you were born with. That's right: FUELLED is here to empower you with recommendations on how to make life-enhancing choices.

Mastering Your Body Comes First

"Take care of your body. It's the only place you have to live."

—Jim Rohn

Now let's step back for a second and look at the bigger picture. Let's look at your life overall and see if we can strengthen your understanding of the previous section.

Psychologist Abraham Maslow, who studied extraordinary people like Albert Einstein and Eleanor Roosevelt, along with the healthiest 1% of a college population, in 1943 laid out a five tier model of human needs, which is often depicted as a pyramid and referred to as "Maslow's Hierarchy of Human Needs." Basically, his theory draws attention to the fact that the most fundamental of human needs, represented by the base of the pyramid, are Physiological needs – those needs related to your physical body as a living organism. Occupying the largest part of the pyramid, those needs are our most basic and necessary. They are absolutely required for human survival and therefore they are the most important and should be met FIRST. Those needs include air, water, food, shelter, warmth (clothing), sex and sleep. In summary, they all relate to our physical health. Our physical health comes first.

It makes sense - if the human body is unwell or broken down or deficient in water, food, sleep, etc, we cannot experience a magnificent quality of life. Not even close! We cannot be all we can be or all that we were brought on this earth to become.

As ancient Greek physician Herophilus said: "When health is absent, wisdom cannot reveal itself, art cannot manifest, strength cannot fight, wealth becomes useless, and intelligence cannot be applied."

You see, Maslow was interested in human potential and how we fulfill that potential. His theory is based on the premise that people are inherently seeking self-fulfillment and the realization of their true potential. He believed that people were motivated to move up to a higher stage in the hierarchy when things were going right in the stage that they were in and, consequently, that their desire for personal growth peaked at the top stage of the pyramid, where experiences of being totally fulfilled and *doing all one is capable of* arise. He called that stage 'Self Actualization.'

A key take away from this model is that Maslow has done the thinking for us and laid out, in order, the various stages in the creation of a *magnificent experience of life*, from the bottom up. His approach

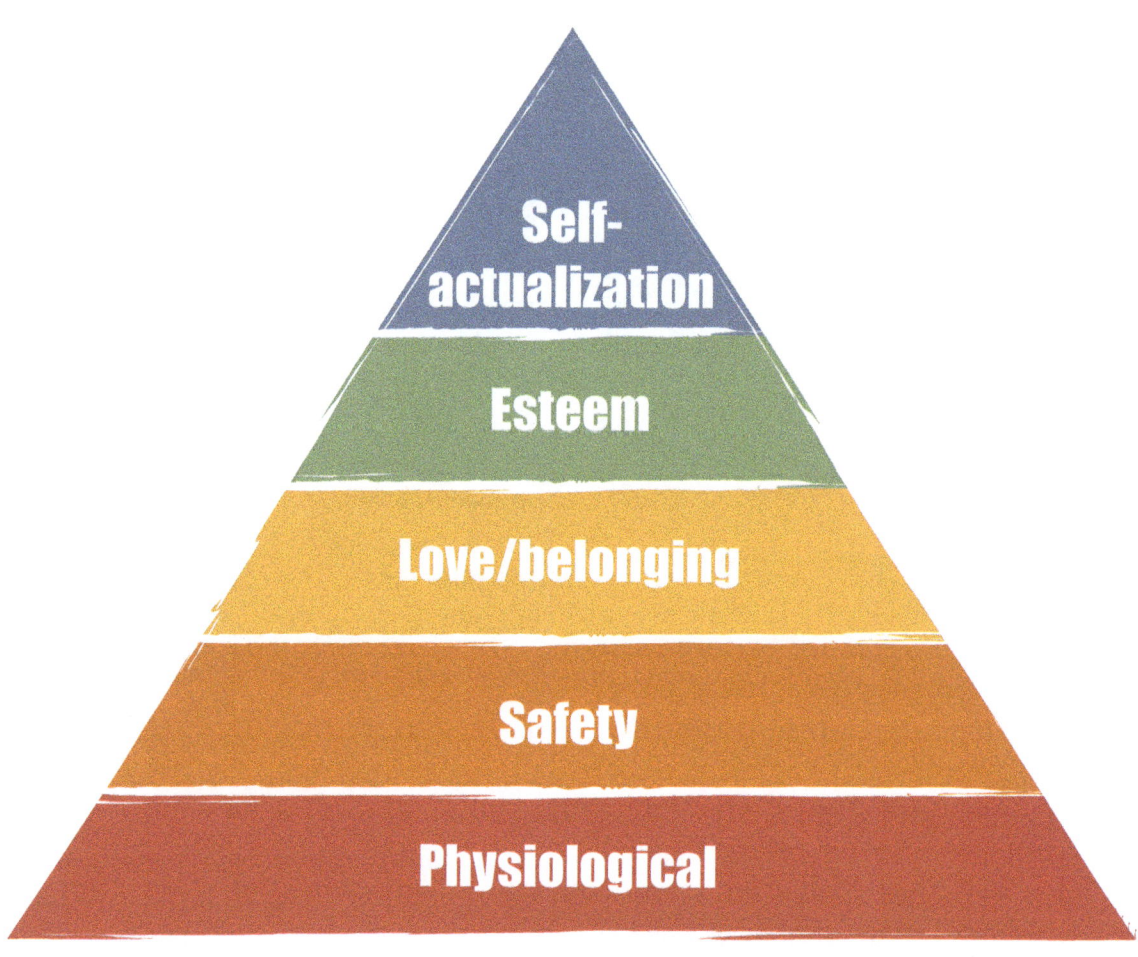

Figure 1-Maslow's human needs, 1943, depicted as a pyramid

allows for an easy appreciation of how important your body's physical needs, like good health, food and water, are to living your very best life.

Tony Robbins, #1 New York Times bestselling author, life and business strategist, philanthropist, and entrepreneur reinforces this message with what he calls a 'Pyramid of Mastery' ("Tie It All Together," 2017). The stages in his pyramid highlight the seven core areas of life that one needs to focus on to create the life they truly deserve. These seven core areas are:

1. Physical body [the foundation]
2. Emotions & Meaning
3. Relationships
4. Time
5. Career & Mission
6. Finances
7. Contribution & Spirituality [the peak]

To me, an extraordinary life comes from a strong commitment to focus on improvement in all seven core areas of life outlined above, and, similarly, on Maslow's pyramid.

However, while all areas of life are very important, there is a step by step journey that creates peak performance and fulfilment. And that journey starts at the base of the pyramid. The foundation of everything you're going to do in your life is your Physical Body. As American entrepreneur, author and motivational speaker Jim Rohn said: "Take care of your body. It's the only place you have to live." It makes sense, right? An amazing life comes from focusing on all areas of both pyramids — but mastering your physical body as a living organism is the *most* crucial part. You really have to master your body.

If you don't master your body – maximize your health, your energy and vitality – all the money, career success, and contribution in the world will not be enjoyed to the absolute fullest. It might even be worthless if you feel sick, tired, overweight and dull, or live in fear of what the doctor might have to tell you on your next visit. It all might not matter if you're:

- Too exhausted to really experience that holiday
- Too tired to play with your children
- Too tired for love or romance
- Too weak for that adventure
- Too unfocused to create goals for yourself
- Too sick to get excited about the next level
- Lacking the vitality to experience joy every day
- Lacking energy to master your emotions so you keep having relationship problems
- Unable to muster up that push to take your business to the next level

You simply cannot experience an extraordinary quality of life without the vehicle that's going to help you create it. I believe that this is exactly what Chopra and Tanzi teach us in *Super Genes*, and what the science of epigenetics is leading us to an understanding of, albeit with more of a focus on human biology than human psychology.

By mastering your physical body — specifically by focusing on better choices that unlock the greatest potential outcomes from your genes, within the cells of your body — you will not only feel more invigorated and energized, you will also have built the foundation for changing your life in profound and extraordinary ways. Mastering your body is the first step in creating the life you really want! And FUELLED is here to present a map of exactly how to do that.

Your Personal Philosophy on Health, Energy and Eating

When was the last time you spent some time thinking about your personal philosophy towards optimal health and energy? We don't often take the time to stop and think.

Take a moment to ask yourself some of these questions:

- What is your definition of optimal health? Is it to be disease-free or something more...?
- Who taught you about optimal health?
- How did you develop your ideas about what heals the body?
- How did you develop your ideas about how to boost your energy? Or what are you doing to boost your energy? Caffeine? Sodas? Energy drinks? Alcohol? Why?
- When you think of achieving your ideal self, do the attitudes 'burden of discipline' and 'wrestling with my willpower' come to mind? If so, why?
- How does your current philosophy or thinking about your health impact how you take care of your body? Is it *helping* — or *hurting*?

Now – really quickly – are these beliefs serving you? Are they empowering you and motivating you to be your most healthy self?

Next, take some time to think about your philosophy on eating and your body.

You can ask yourself these questions:

- Do you think food is *for you* or *against you*? Why?
- Do you think that healthy food tastes disgusting? Why?
- When you think about being on a diet to lose weight, how does that make you feel about eating? How does it make you feel about your body? Your life?
- What are your beliefs surrounding how to shed excess weight? Where did those come from?

- Do you feel that sustained weight loss and enhanced energy for the long term is always about trying hard? If so, why?

Now – really quickly – are these beliefs serving you? Are they empowering you and motivating you to be your most healthy self?

Few people take the time to investigate where their current philosophies come from, meanwhile, these beliefs and the stories behind them (that we tell ourselves) are driving our decisions about health, eating and energy every single day of our lives. What I mean to say is that many of us have negative or limiting beliefs about our bodies and our health. We tell ourselves that losing weight is hard. We believe that eating healthy is not easy. We think, I don't have the time or energy right now to improve my health; it's too much work.

These hard-wired beliefs only make it more difficult for us to take charge of our health, bodies and destiny. Until something shakes us up. A new idea, an approach, a theory, a book. Hopefully, that *something* provides us with more empowering beliefs than the ones we held before.

Think about it. What type of transformation could you experience in your life if you let go of your old beliefs about your body, food, energy and your capacity for outstanding health and took on a new perspective that expanded your choices, options and outlook?

What if you decided today that you were finally going to unlock the power of true **FUEL = Food Unleashing Energy for Life**? Isn't it time you made full use of the capacity within you?

What the Body Needs to Stay Healthy

Here's what you really need to know about what your body needs so that you can FUEL it properly.

The Physical Body's Essential Needs

1. Fresh Air, Water and Light
2. Green Foods and Drinks
3. Essential Fatty Acids
4. Protein (Essential Amino Acids)
5. Phytonutrients
6. Vitamins
7. Enzymes
8. Minerals
9. Fibre
10. Antioxidants
11. Friendly Micro-Organisms

This list is your new guidepost for understanding what your body's needs are, and how to make sure you're getting all of these on a regular or daily basis. Let me explain them.

Fresh Air, Water and Light — These are relatively self-explanatory. Of course you need fresh air, water and sunshine to live! However, hydration is a key part of FUELLING your body everyday. Check out the **Wonders of Water** section for more information.

Green Foods and Drinks — Green foods, like kale, spinach and broccoli, contain an abundance of nutrients and vitamins necessary for optimal health. Cruciferous vegetables (like broccoli) are very high in vitamin A, vitamin C, folic acid and fibre. Spinach is high in calcium, iron, magnesium, potassium, vitamin A and folic acid. Greens foods are often low in calories but packed with nutrients, making them nutritiously-dense foods. These will be covered in depth in this book.

Essential Fatty Acids (EFAs) — Fatty acids that your body cannot produce on its own, making them essential to your diet. The two primary EFAs are omega-6 and omega-3. Check out the **Healthy (and Downright Essential) Fats and Oils** section for more information.

Protein (Essential Amino Acids) — Amino acids cannot be made in the body, so we must get them from our diet. There are 9 essential amino acids that humans cannot produce, making it necessary that we eat foods that contain them. These are found in plant and animal protein. These are:

1. Histidine
2. Isoleucine
3. Leucine
4. Lysine
5. Methionine
6. Phenylalanine
7. Threonine
8. Tryptophan
9. Valine

Learn more in the **Perfect Protein** section of this book.

Phytonutrients or Phytochemicals — The natural chemicals found in plant foods, like fruits and vegetables, whole grains, nuts, beans and herbal tea. Phytonutrients like Resveratrol can help your body prevent disease. More information can be found further in this book.

Vitamins — Vital nutrients that your body need to maintain optimal health. Vitamins help your body grow and develop normally. Each vitamin performs a different function in the body, so it's important to make sure that you have all the vitamins in your diet. The essential vitamins that your body needs are:

- Vitamin A
- Vitamin C

- Vitamin D
- Vitamin E
- Vitamin K
- B vitamins

Enzymes — These can generally be broken down into 3 groups: metabolic enzymes, digestive enzymes and food enzymes. All play a crucial role in your health, metabolism and digestion.

Minerals — There are two types of minerals: macrominerals and trace minerals. You need larger amounts of macrominerals, like calcium, magnesium, and potassium. Trace minerals you need in smaller amounts, and include iron and zinc.

Fibre — Promotes digestion and is crucial for optimal health. Dietary fibre, found primarily in fruits, vegetables, whole grains and legumes, can help you maintain a healthy weight, improve digestion and lower your risk of diabetes and heart disease.

Antioxidants — Protect the body from damage and disease. They do so by stopping free radicals, the unstable molecules that steal from healthy cells in your body and cause damaging changes. Some examples of antioxidants include beta-carotene and selenium. The best sources are fruits and vegetables. Many antioxidants are also classified as phytonutrients.

Friendly Micro-Organisms — Friendly bacteria that fight against harmful, disease-causing bacteria in the body. We all have trillions of bacteria living in our intestines and there is an increasing body of research that highlights the impact that imbalanced gut bacteria may have on our health, including, but not restricted to, digestive issues and weakened immunity. Balancing your gut bacteria with beneficial high quality probiotic supplements, fermented foods and a balanced diet will help keep these micro-organisms in check.

Let's RAISE THE BAR On What You Expect Food Can Do For You

A major component of the FUELLED philosophy is *Raising the Bar* on what you expect food can do for you. This might sound wild but have you ever looked at your plate or glass and thought: Food — what have you done for me lately?

It's time to look at food differently. It's time to expect so much more. Food is now a powerful FUEL for you to use to reach your optimal level of health — and then to *power* you to the next level in your career, your relationships and your spiritual, emotional and mental wellbeing.

Raising the Bar is about understanding that the food on your plate can be powerful and potent — it's about so much more than filling your cravings and hunger so that they go away. It's about looking at your plate, at your food, at those carrots, that fish, that oil and that pressed vegetable juice and seeing in it the power to harness the best from your genes. To activate an enormous amount of untapped potential. To optimize your cellular health and therefore your body's daily functioning to create outstanding outcomes for yourself. That's what *Raising the Bar* on what you expect your food to do for you is all about. And only the *best* outcomes come from the *best* foods. The foods you choose to eat — specifically if you choose green, leafy vegetables and nutrient-dense foods — have a direct impact on your gene expression and your potential for a healthy, bright, vibrant life. Remember, if we want an extraordinary quality of life, we better have an extraordinary cell life.

When you choose to *Raise the Bar* on what food can do for you, you are making a profound shift in your mindset. You now understand the impact it can have on you. Starting today, try looking at food differently. Expect more. So much more. *Raise the Bar* on food to achieve optimal health long-term.

The FUELLED Food Pyramid

So let's make this visual and see how it translates into REAL FOOD. Here's a pyramid. We have all encountered food pyramids, plates etc. This is a very modern one that provides a map for a healthier and more vital life than you could ever have imagined.

Like a traditional food pyramid, the base - that's the biggest part - shows what you should consume in the largest quantities — the first 3 rungs are all plant based, life-giving, water-rich foods like green vegetables and their juices, other colourful vegetables and fruits. Some examples of all of these include: organic green vegetables like spinach, kale, lettuce, collard greens, leeks, parsley, cucumber, broccoli, watercress, cabbage, zucchini, green bell peppers, green beans, etc., and their fresh-pressed or blended juices (where applicable); colourful vegetables like pumpkin, onions, carrots, beets, sweet potatoes, mushrooms, eggplant, bell peppers, parsnips, radishes, fennel, cauliflower, and their fresh-pressed or blended juices; and fruits like lemons, grapefruits, apples, berries, bananas, pineapples, plums, papaya, kiwi, pears, watermelon, rhubarb, etc., and their fresh-pressed or blended juices. However, unlike a traditional food pyramid, this one

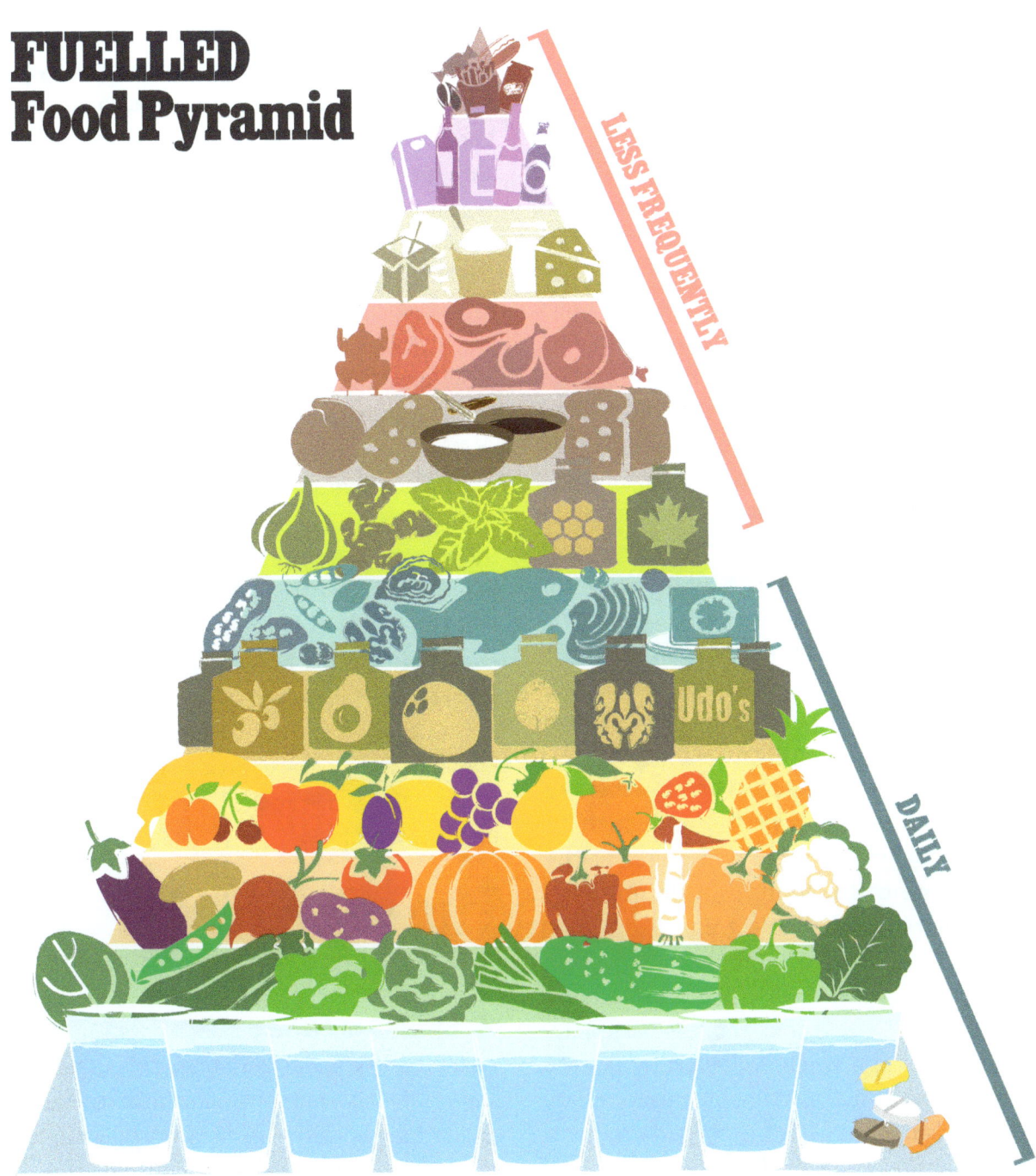

has the base that I just described standing on top of 8 glasses of fresh, filtered, pure water — an absolute essential in your daily journey towards optimal health. Alongside that stand 4 supplements and those would be your daily high-quality multivitamin, probiotic, fish oil or vegan alternative, and vitamin D3.

Moving up from the vegetables and fruits, the FUELLED pyramid recommends consuming healthy fats and oils every single day, like those found in organic extra virgin olive oil, flaxseed oil or flaxseeds, hempseed oil or hempseeds, Udo's Choice Oil, avocado oil, and coconut oil. That's right folks: bring fats back to the table! Then, in smaller portions but still daily and at every meal, come plant-based proteins like those found in nuts and nut butters (excluding peanuts), seeds like hempseeds and chia seeds, pumpkin seeds, sunflower seeds and beans, lentils etc., and seafood like deep sea fish, oysters, clams and mussels.

Those are followed by herbs, fermented foods and healthy sweeteners, which all provide health benefits and enhance the flavour of healthy foods, but do not have to be eaten daily. Whole grains like brown rice, quinoa and teff (an Ethiopian grain that is extraordinarily high in iron) should be eaten in smaller portions and less frequently throughout the week, followed by quality, organic, grass-fed, sustainably raised meats like chicken, turkey, beef, buffalo, duck, lamb, and goat (but not including pork).

And moving up towards the top — and the top is what you should have the least of — you see dairy products including yogurt, cheese, ice cream, whipped cream, butter, milk; followed by juice, wine and beer and then at the very top: highly processed, canned and pre-packaged foods, a "food group" literally labeled here as "JUNK" because companies use chemicals to preserve, colour, and flavour-up these foods.

JUNK includes all refined carbohydrates, most store-bought breads, cakes, frozen pizza, chips, instant dinners, anything dyed an unnatural colour, boxed cereals and commercially produced granola, coffee, sugar, candy bars, sodas, most alcohol, processed meats like deli meats, French fries, and most fast food. These should be eaten in very limited amounts. See **The 90/10 Rule for Success** section that comes later in the book to learn how to best incorporate these into your life.

Overall, it is clear to see that the point is eliminating sugary, processed foods and other JUNK while focusing on organic, real, unprocessed foods.

The Wonders of Water

Water is an essential component of our health and vitality. It is a nutrient found in foods, liquids and in its own form (pure water). Examples of water sources include pure, filtered or spring water; coconut water; herbal teas like chamomile, peppermint, rosehip, hibiscus, apple, licorice, ginger tea, etc.; fruits like watermelon, oranges, lemons, pineapples, apples and grapes; vegetables like lettuce, broccoli, carrots and beets; green juices, smoothies, fruit juices and, of course, ice.

Water is a major component of all living matter and the human body is composed of about 60% water. We lose water continuously throughout the day through breathing, sweating, urinating and defecating and that water loss varies based on environment (hot, humid or dry, cold climates or higher/lower altitudes) and activity level.

What's absolutely certain is that our water loss needs to be replenished or we become dehydrated. Symptoms of dehydration range from dry mouth and headaches to stress, allergies, weight gain, and other more serious states of *dis-ease* (Batmanghelidj, 2003). Next time you have a headache, try fully hydrating yourself before you do anything else.

The benefits of consuming plenty of water every single day are far reaching and cannot be underestimated.

STOP guzzling water with every meal! Yes, you read that correctly, and, yes, I know how radical and unconventional it sounds. Water is served at every restaurant, with every meal. Here's the thing: When you are eating, you want all your energy directed at breaking down food so your body can easily assimilate the nutrients and eliminate waste. So, it is best if you do not drink water or liquids, especially ice cold ones, while eating your meals. Drink water or any liquid at least 20 minutes before and at least 20 minutes after your meals (ideally an hour) – but not during. The reason for that is that drinking liquids during your meal dilutes your naturally occurring digestive enzymes and stomach acids, which makes it harder to break down food. This means that you are actually complicating things for your stomach and intestines and not deriving the maximum nourishment from all the good foods you're eating. The best time to hydrate your body is between meals – so pay close attention to staying hydrated and drinking your liquids in the time you have between breakfast, lunch and dinner. And if you feel that you need the extra liquids to process the food in your mouth, then it's time to start chewing properly and creating the saliva necessary to moisten the foods and swallow them comfortably. If you still feel that you need to drink something, then I highly recommend sipping on an herbal tea like peppermint, ginger or chamomile or room temperature water with lemon in it, which are easier on the system and may assist digestion.

But HOLD ON... Don't Drink Liquids With Your Meals!

EDUCATE

Water:

- Increases energy and relieves fatigue
- Promotes weight loss and helps us feel satiated
- Maintains our balance of body fluids
- Flushes out toxins, cleansing and detoxifying our system
- Combats muscle fatigue and cramping
- Improves the look, feel and health of our skin
- Maintains regular bowel function
- Boosts our immune system
- Is a natural headache remedy
- And much more…

One thing is for sure: Do not miss out on one of the easiest ways to FUEL your body!

Focusing on YOUR FOUNDATION

Let's explore the key sections of the FUELLED pyramid starting with the foundation. These foods are plant-based nutrient powerhouses that pack large doses of your body's vital needs. They totally FUEL your cells by providing maximum nourishment. That's because they contain "phytonutrients" (sometimes referred to as "phytochemicals") which is something you do not want to miss out on *ever*. The prefix "phyto" comes from the Greek word for plant, and it's used because phytonutrients are obtained only from plants. Each plant contains tens of thousands of these phytonutrients which it developed to protect itself from the environment. They also cause the plant to have its unique flavour, colour and smell, and they have a very positive effect on us when we eat them. When you focus on eating these plant-based nutrient powerhouses, you create an environment that continually produces, nurtures, strengthens and reinforces vital, healthy and strong cells. And, in case you were wondering, you cannot gain the same effect from taking a supplement.

That means eat lots of water-rich, fresh, alive, (organic wherever possible) green foods like:

- Kale
- Spinach
- Collard Greens
- Swiss Chard
- Parsley
- Broccoli rabe
- Cucumber
- Asparagus
- Leeks
- Kohlrabi
- Broccoli
- Mustard greens
- Scallions
- Watercress
- Zucchini

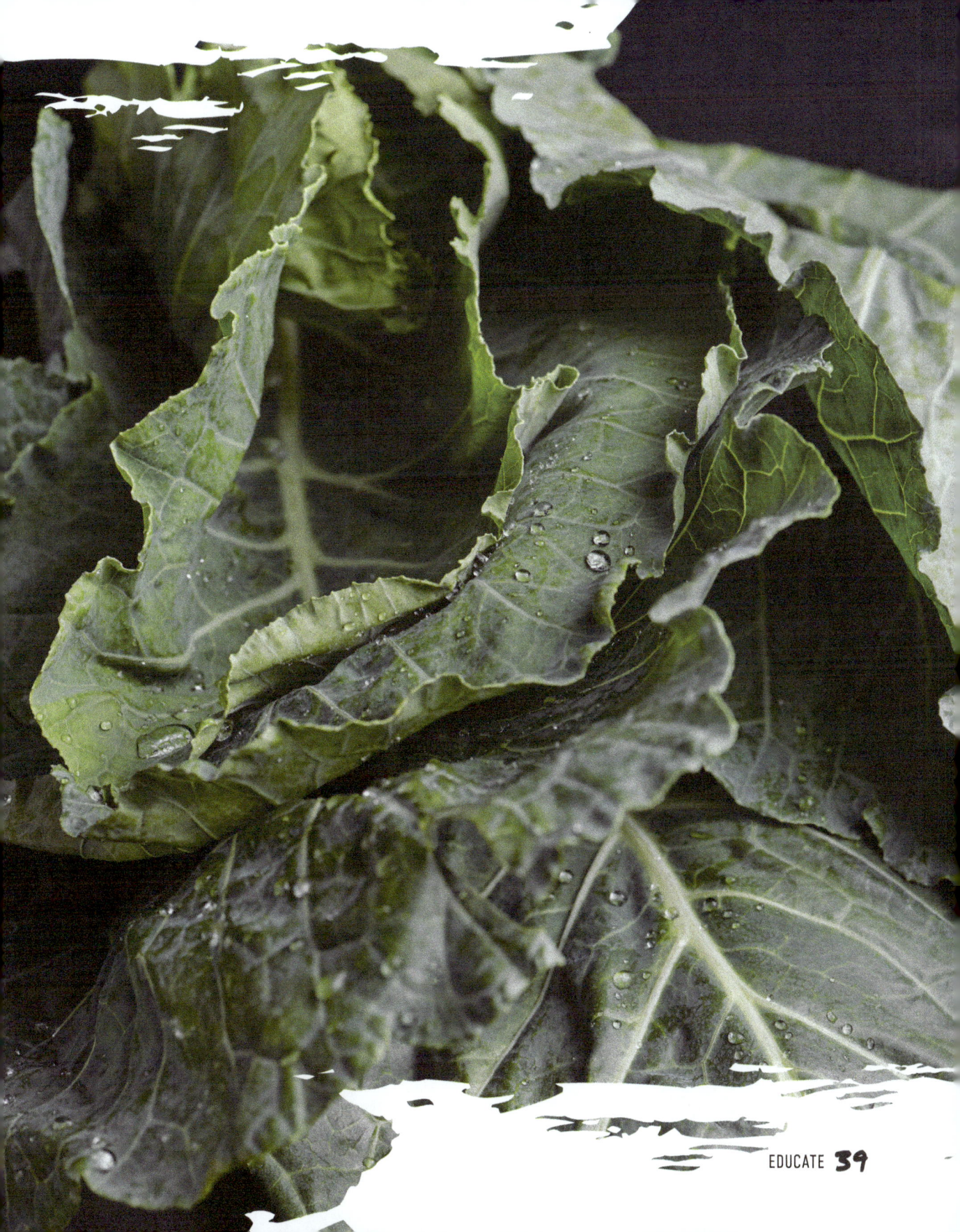

- Lettuce – Red, Green Leaf, Boston, Romaine, Butter
- Green beans
- Green peas
- Cabbage
- Brussels sprouts
- Arugula (or "Rocket")
- Bok choy
- Green bell peppers
- Beet greens
- Wheatgrass (and Spirulina and Chlorella)
- Superfood green drinks
- And many more…

They provide healthy nutrients that FUEL your cells and purify and cleanse your body. They are simply life-giving.

And also eat plenty of colourful raw, roasted or cooked (organic wherever possible) vegetables like:

- Beets – all colours
- Carrots – all colours
- Pumpkin and squash – all types
- Cabbage – red, green, all types and colours
- Okra
- Onions – all types and colours
- Bell peppers – all colours
- Sweet potatoes and yams
- Radishes – all types
- Fennel
- Cauliflower
- Mushrooms – all types
- Eggplant – all types
- Parsnips
- Rutabaga
- Turnips
- And many more…

Getting a variety of colours in your daily FUEL is the best way forward. Certain colours of food indicate an abundance of specific nutrients like vitamin A, B, C and K. Dazzle and honour yourself with a plate or bowl filled with purple, orange, red, yellow, green and white vegetables. Go ahead and learn a bit more about the nutritional value of the foods you want to try and how they compare to the things you already eat. Just by keeping it colourful, you'll ensure that you're getting a range of amazing nutrients to propel yourself forward every single day.

Also, if you suffer from a sweet tooth for candy, cakes and cookies – a great tip is to ensure you're eating sweet vegetables often, like carrots, pumpkin, beets, onions (so sweet when grilled or pan fried), and sweet potatoes, as they will satisfy sugar cravings. You would be surprised how much you can curb sugar cravings for unhealthy sweets like ice cream or candy bars just by adding some roasted sweet potatoes, roasted pumpkin or grilled onions to your day.

And also fresh, raw, organic (if possible) fruit like:

- Apples
- Grapefruit, oranges, lemons, limes and other citrus fruit
- Pineapple

Phytonutrient Colour Wheel

- Blueberries, raspberries, blackberries, strawberries, gooseberries
- Bananas
- Coconuts
- Plums
- Pears
- Cherries
- Peaches, nectarines
- Black and red currants
- Mangoes
- Pomegranates
- Kiwis
- Avocados (yes, this is technically a fruit)
- Watermelon
- Passion fruit
- Papaya
- Cherimoya
- Lychee
- Rhubarb
- Acai and Goji berries (even dried)
- And many more...

Now, I'm sure that there are no surprises here with any of these lists of foundational foods. It's very likely that you already knew that every one of these was what your mom would say were "good for you." But come on, when you hear the word "Broccoli" what is the first thing that comes to your mind? Is it "Ew!!!" or "Do I have to...?" If so, that's probably because you've never had broccoli done right. I'm not kidding. That's why I have a chapter later in this book that explains how incredibly easy it is to create delicious roasted vegetables — like perfect roasted broccoli — that are universally pleasurable to eat and will make you change your mind forever about this green vegetable and others. To be honest, it's because so many of us have had absolutely horrific experiences — *feel your stomach turning?* — or just downright boring experiences — *feel like yawning?* or *that's just not delicious, thank you* — eating vegetables like beets, Brussels sprouts, kale, spinach and cabbage that I created a Real Food How-To Recipe Guide in Part 3: *Transform* that provides directions for taking any of these foods and making them absolutely delicious to eat for breakfast, lunch, dinner or anything in between.

I have a passion for food. I've been cooking for 20 years and, in that time, I've learned how to make *all* foods tasty. That's the goal. To create delicious and nourishing food. I have spent years thinking about how I can deliver food that will actually benefit whomever eats it. That will actually FUEL their body. And now I'm passing that onto you.

If you want to take it one step further, I will let you in on a secret. The majority of the foods in the foundation of the FUELLED Food Pyramid are today considered "Superfoods." *A Superfood is a non-scientific term but it describes a food that contains extraordinary nutritional potency. They're nutrient powerhouses that pack large doses of antioxidants, vitamins, minerals, etc. And the benefits of eating them are so far-reaching, far beyond normal food.* My father likes to refer to them as "Super – *natural* – foods." There's an energetic power to these foods. It may not be a legitimate legal, medical or scientific term but if you are what you eat then I'd prefer, above anything else, to be a Superfood. A nutrient powerhouse. A powerful protector and healer. A rich source of life energy. A food that FUELs.

Organic or Conventional? That is the Question.

Whether to buy organic or non-organic fruits and vegetables is a very important decision, and it's actually much easier to know what to do than you might think. And...guess what? You really don't have to buy everything organic.

Lucky for us, there is a non-profit, non-partisan organization that is dedicated to protecting human health and the environment that we can turn to to help us answer this question in a practical way. This organization is called The Environmental Working Group, or EWG. Their website is www.ewg.org and their mission is to "empower people to live healthier lives in a healthier environment." Their breakthrough research is aimed at connecting people and the environment in an intimate way – they evaluate the safety of personal care products, tap water, home cleaning products, foods and more. As relates to food, they produce a very popular annual guide that you need to know about – EWG's Shopper's Guide to Pesticides in Produce. And from that guide, they have created 2 shortlists that cover the best and worst of what you need to know about produce this year, creatively named "The Dirty Dozen" and "The Clean Fifteen." These lists tell you exactly what they sound like they would: The Dirty Dozen tells you which non-organic fruits and vegetables are the most covered in pesticide residue and The Clean Fifteen tells you which non-organic fruits and vegetables are the "cleanest" or least covered in harmful pesticide residues. Basically, having these lists with you when you go to buy groceries (and you can get free wallet-size lists on their website) helps you avoid The Dirty Dozen – buy organic ONLY for those items. Try not to buy conventional fruits and vegetables covered in harmful chemicals. No matter how well you wash them, for those dirtiest fruits and vegetables, the residues are really bad. So, again, that's where you want to splurge and buy organic. However, choose non-organic items from the Clean Fifteen List. That's right – For the Clean Fifteen, you do not need to splurge on organic. Buy conventional there. See how easy that is? Done.

EWG's 2017 Dirty 12™

1. STRAWBERRIES
2. SPINACH
3. NECTARINES
4. APPLES
5. PEACHES
6. PEARS
7. CHERRIES
8. GRAPES
9. CELERY
10. TOMATOES
11. SWEET BELL PEPPERS
12. POTATOES

Copyright © Environmental Working Group, www.ewg.org. Reproduced with permission.

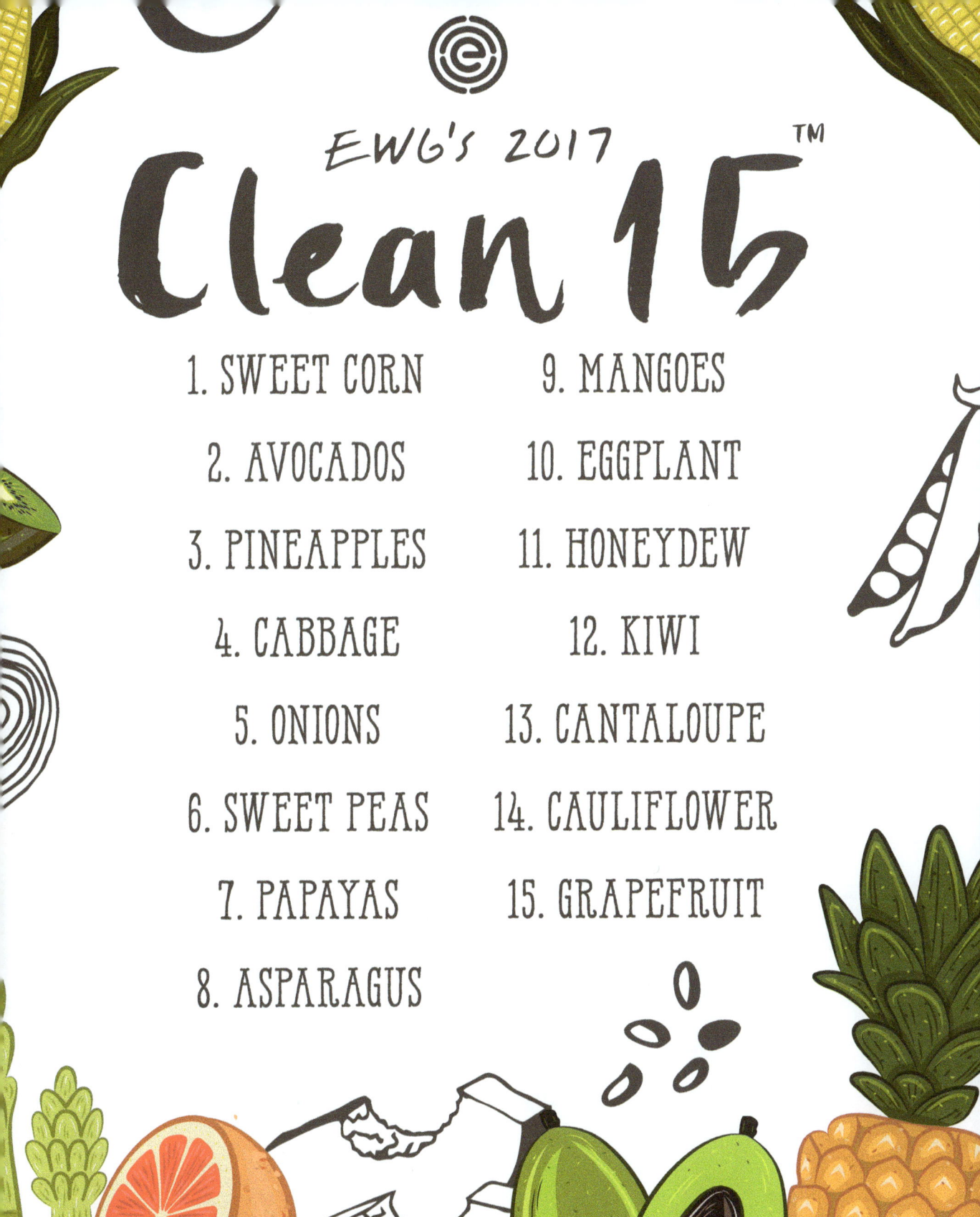

Check the PLU Code

PLU codes or Price Look-Up codes have been used by supermarkets for over 30 years to make check-out and inventory control easier, faster and more accurate. They are assigned to fruits and vegetables following a review process conducted by the International Federation for Produce Standards (IFPS). Why do you need to know this? Because, even though they are not intended to convey information to consumers, a quick glance at a code can help you confirm a few key details.

5-DIGIT CODE
BEGINNING WITH 9

▼

ORGANIC

94153

4-DIGIT CODE
BEGINNING WITH 3 OR 4

▼

CONVENTIONALY GROWN

3626

5-DIGIT CODE
THAT STARTS WITH 8

Previously designated to identify GMO produce items but IFPS is transitioning away from that to open up all the '8' prefix codes to accommodate an increase in varieties of fresh produce items that are both conventionally grown and organically grown as they enter the market. According to IFPS, the '8' prefix was not being used at retail and so removing the GMO designation opens up 1,000 additional codes. (It is widely believed that GMO produce sellers were concerned their sales would drop if consumers saw the '8' prefix, so they were utilizing the '3' or '4' codes for conventional produce to mark their items).

Therefore, the leading digit '8' will have no significance soon.

However, the 83000 series will be used to assign codes for conventionally grown produce items and the 84000 series will be used to identify the corresponding organic item

Healthy (and Downright Essential) Fats and Oils

"It's not FATS that make you FAT"
– Udo Erasmus

If you want to be FUELLED, you need to get educated and get real about FAT. You might have already known to eat your spinach and broccoli but eating your essential fats and oils might be new. Before diving into the types and sources, I'm going to address a major roadblock that arises for most people in this area: The erroneous myth that fat is fattening.

Chances are that you or someone you know thinks that eating fat will make you fat. That's because we live in a society where, in recent history, since the 1980's, (United States Federal Government, 1980), we were constantly bombarded with messages telling us to cut fat entirely out of our diet. Remember all the fat-free cookies, salad dressings, soups, sauces, etc.? And there is still so much conflicting information out there. For instance, on June 15, 2017, the American Heart Association released a report stating that coconut oil is not good for you because of the saturated fat content (Sacks, et al.) while numerous other studies show that virgin coconut oil is an extremely healthy saturated fat that heals the body. What's a person to do?

Fats in general have gotten a bad rap in our "heart-healthy" and fat-obsessed diet culture. I'm here to tell you that that concept is old science and simply untrue. It's time for everyone to get real about fat. Fat is an excellent FUEL for your body and your brain, when chosen correctly. So it is time to re-examine your relationship with fats and oils and what they can do for you. You need to readjust your mindset.

You have got to be sure you are getting the quality fats that your body needs from your diet. Lack of high-quality fat in the diet is linked to poor skin health, amenorrhea, hormonal imbalance, cravings you can't kick, poorer brain function, moodiness and a slew of other health issues. Your body needs to take in essential fats, known as omega 3 and omega 6 fatty acids. What "essential fats" means is that your body does not produce these essential nutrients on its own but they are crucial building blocks for life and are vital to your well-being. So you need to get them from the foods you eat.

The key takeaway is that not all fats are created equally and not all affect the body in the same way.

Here's what you need to know about the Power of Healthy and Essential Fats and Oils (aka Essential Fatty Acids):

There are basically 2 types of fats: Fats that heal and fats that kill (Erasmus, 1998)

EDUCATE

Fats that Heal — These are health promoting fats and oils

- Essential fats are healthy or healing fats that your body cannot make itself but every cell in the body requires them to function and so must obtain them from foods
- The most important are omega 3 and omega 6 essential fatty acids (EFAs). These are found within what are known as "unsaturated fats" but I won't get further into the science of it to keep it as simple as possible
- Omega 3 and 6 essential fatty acids are required building blocks of life and your health will decline if you are deficient in them, but if you start to take them then the symptoms reverse because your body knows what to do with these nutrients right away
- People today are generally deficient in omega 3 and too high in omega 6
- Too much omega 6 is linked to inflammation and a decline in health
- The ideal ratio of omega 6 to omega 3 is somewhere between 1:1 and 4:1, which is generally represented in the list of healthy fats that follows. Do not stress about this ratio, just try to get the healthiest fats you can into your body every single day
- There are also healthy saturated fats such as coconut oil

The role omega 3 and omega 6 essential fats and oils play in your body are that they:

- Provide building blocks for cell membranes
- Raise metabolism
- Aid in digestion
- Aid in the production of hormones, including sex hormones testosterone and estrogen
- Reduce inflammation
- Protect our body by buffering and neutralizing acids
- Provide lubrication in our body so that our cells are free to move
- Improve and heal skin conditions
- Elevate our mood, lift depression and improve our ability to deal with stress
- Stabilize the heartbeat
- Lower our risk of heart disease
- Prevent and reverse degenerative diseases
- Increase bone building properties
- Are an antioxidant powerhouse and play a role in anti-aging
- The brain needs them to function optimally — they boost our brain power
- Increase energy
- Help our body absorb vitamins A, D, E and K
- Help our body absorb minerals such as calcium
- Fat is satiating, leaving us feeling full and satisfied. It curbs cravings.

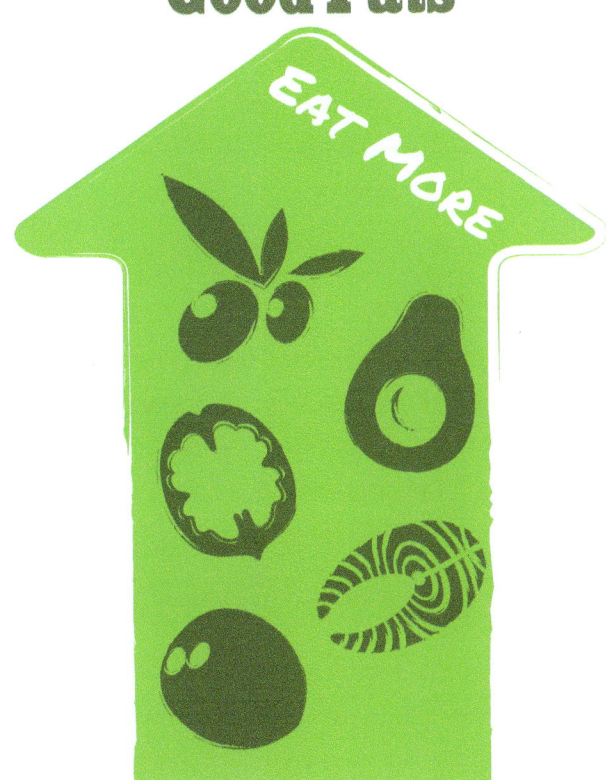 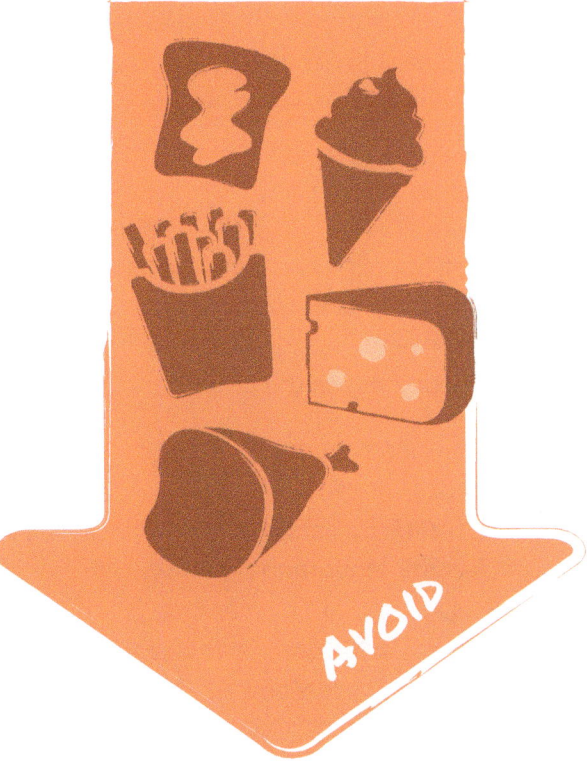

Talk about having beneficial, life-extending, age-defying properties! These essential fats and oils are the complete opposite of being harmful and fattening to our body.

And here's some more great news: They're DELICIOUS!

The best natural sources are (in no particular order):

- Udo's Oil DHA 3-6-9 Blend
- Hempseeds or hempseed oil
- Flaxseeds (ground) or flaxseed oil
- Avocados
- Fish oil supplements
- Fat off healthy, fatty fish, such as herring, sardines, mackerel, wild salmon and trout
- Extra virgin olive oil
- Nuts and seeds, nut butter or seed butter (walnuts, pumpkin seeds, sesame seeds, sunflower seeds)
- Virgin coconut oil (which is actually a healthy saturated fat)

EDUCATE

It is important to note that you cannot fry most of the healthy essential fats and oils such as flaxseed, hempseed and Udo's Oil because they lose a lot of their nutritional potency when heated. In order to take in the most benefits from them, they must be consumed raw, cold-pressed and as fresh as possible. Keep them refrigerated at all times. Use different oils for frying, roasting, or any other cooking, such as avocado oil, grapeseed or olive oil.

Some health risks associated with diets low in these good fats, on the other hand, include:

- Poor brain function
- Compromised heart health
- Hormone imbalances and the risk of infertility in women
- Weight gain and overeating
- Higher risk for depression and anxiety
- Gut related problems

Fats that Kill — These are fats and oils that damage human health

Some examples of unhealthy fats and oils include:

- Industrially processed and refined fats found in boxed foods and most restaurant foods (all of the below)
- Trans fats ("hydrogenated oils") – check all your food labels if you eat boxed foods!
- Margarine
- Mayonnaise
- Pork lard
- Industrially proceeded shortening like Crisco – which is really hydrogenated cottonseed and/or soybean oil
- Industrial seed oils, also known as "vegetable oils" (ex. canola oil, soybean, peanut, safflower, sunflower, cottonseed oil, which are entirely too high in omega 6's and cause chronic inflammation)
- Corn oil

If you could see it on a spectrum, it might make a lot more sense: on the one side you know that bacon isn't a health food, but on the other side you know that an avocado is a health food. When you look at that spectrum, think about the fats that you're eating...where do those lie?

Basically, I want you to *Raise the Bar* on what healthy fats can do for you. So, if you're still living in the low-fat, no-fat mentality of weight loss, weigh maintenance or health, if anything "high-fat" still sets off alarm bells and raises concerns about packing on the pounds then it's time to reassess and re-evaluate those notions and beliefs and readjust your mindset. It's time to get real about fat. Fat is excellent FUEL for your brain and for your body. But not all fats are the same so I have outlined the best sources of these life-giving vital nutrients. I would strongly encourage you to increase your intake of these wonderful, healthy and essential fats in your diet.

Perfect Proteins

Protein is essential to a healthy diet. It is made up of nature's little chemical rock stars called amino acids. *Aminos* form the foundation for many of our cells, tissues and muscles — they are crucial to our overall cellular fitness. When we eat foods that contain protein, the amino acids are broken down during digestion and absorbed into our cells and muscles. Taken in the right quantities, protein can repair, restore and build our muscles and other tissues. And although our bodies naturally produce some of the amino acids that create protein,

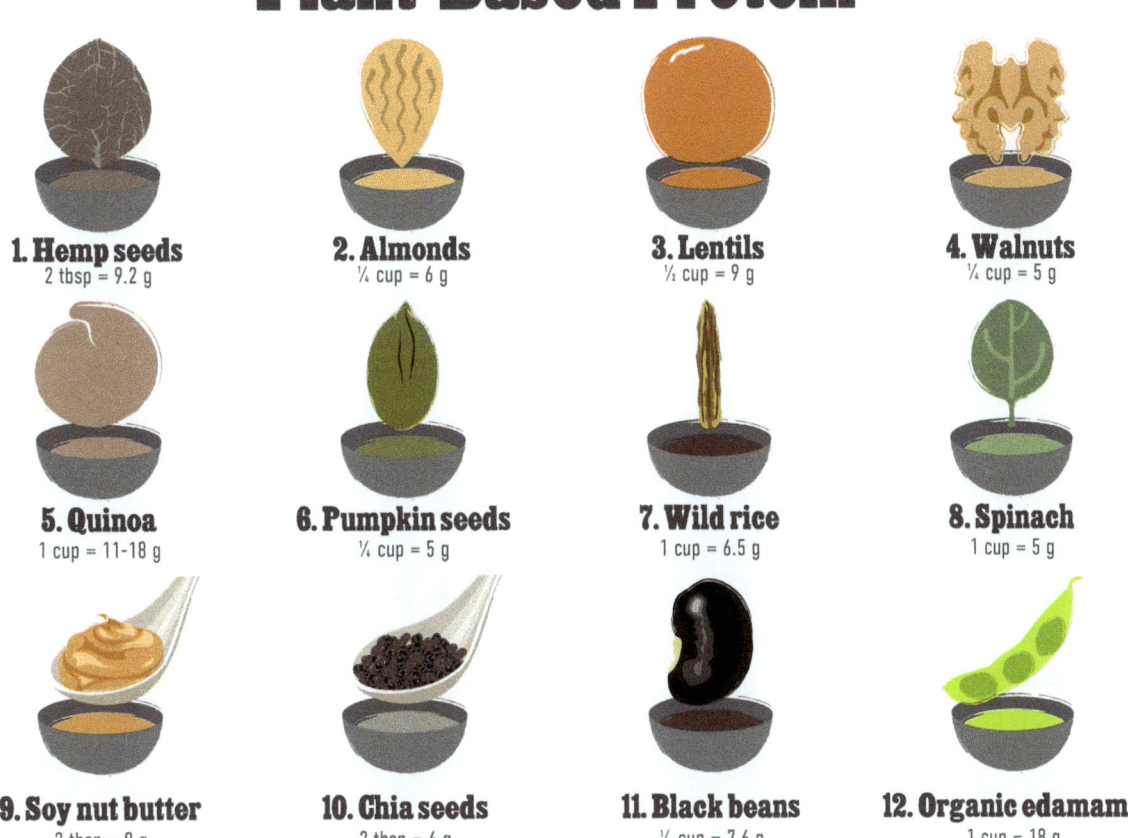

12 Great Sources of Plant-Based Protein

1. **Hemp seeds** — 2 tbsp = 9.2 g
2. **Almonds** — ¼ cup = 6 g
3. **Lentils** — ½ cup = 9 g
4. **Walnuts** — ¼ cup = 5 g
5. **Quinoa** — 1 cup = 11-18 g
6. **Pumpkin seeds** — ¼ cup = 5 g
7. **Wild rice** — 1 cup = 6.5 g
8. **Spinach** — 1 cup = 5 g
9. **Soy nut butter** — 2 tbsp = 9 g
10. **Chia seeds** — 2 tbsp = 6 g
11. **Black beans** — ½ cup = 7.6 g
12. **Organic edamame** — 1 cup = 18 g

diets containing protein are necessary to supplement our natural stores so that our body can reach its greatest potential.

The FUELLED Pyramid recommends eating plant-based protein at every meal and seafood as often as you're able to.

Plant Protein

Plant-based protein sounds like a new thing but it really isn't. You've been eating plant-based protein your entire life and probably didn't know it.

The infographic on the previous page shows 12 great sources of plant-based protein as well as how much protein they provide per serving.

The benefits of eating plant-based protein are numerous. Plant-based diets reduce the risk of heart disease, cancer and other health problems; they contain an abundance of good-for-you nutrients; they are more environmentally sustainable than animal protein as they use fewer resources to produce; they don't harm animals; and plant-based diets are free of dairy allergens and animal by-products. Nuts, seeds, nut butters, quinoa, wild rice, beans, lentils and certain vegetables are also some of nature's treasures. They are nutrient powerhouses, loaded with disease-fighting phytonutrients, cholesterol-lowering fibre and are naturally low in sodium. They also keep you feeling full, reducing the need to overeat or snack on unhealthy foods. Eating plant protein every single day gives you a nutritional advantage.

Seafood

Numerous studies have validated the health benefits of seafood, especially high quality, wild-caught fish. That said, seafood is a term that encompasses fish and shellfish — so everything from canned tuna to fresh tilapia to lobster is considered "seafood." So whether or not you live by the ocean, knowing what you consume from the ocean is more important than ever. When it comes to seafood, knowledge is power. Selecting and eating the right seafood can leave your body FUELLED, as it boosts your energy and immune system. However, it's now more important than ever to understand the types of seafood that you should avoid. But first, let's start with the amazing benefits of a seafood-rich diet.

Seafood Benefits: High Protein, Low Calorie

Fish, such as Wild Alaskan Salmon, are a terrific source of natural protein. For example, a 100 gram portion of King or Sockeye (Red) Alaskan salmon contains approximately 20 grams of protein for only 220-230 calories (USDA, 2017b). Compare that to a major US peanut butter brand, where the same portion would provide just over 20 grams of protein for 618 calories (USDA, 2017d). That's three times the calories for the same amount of protein!

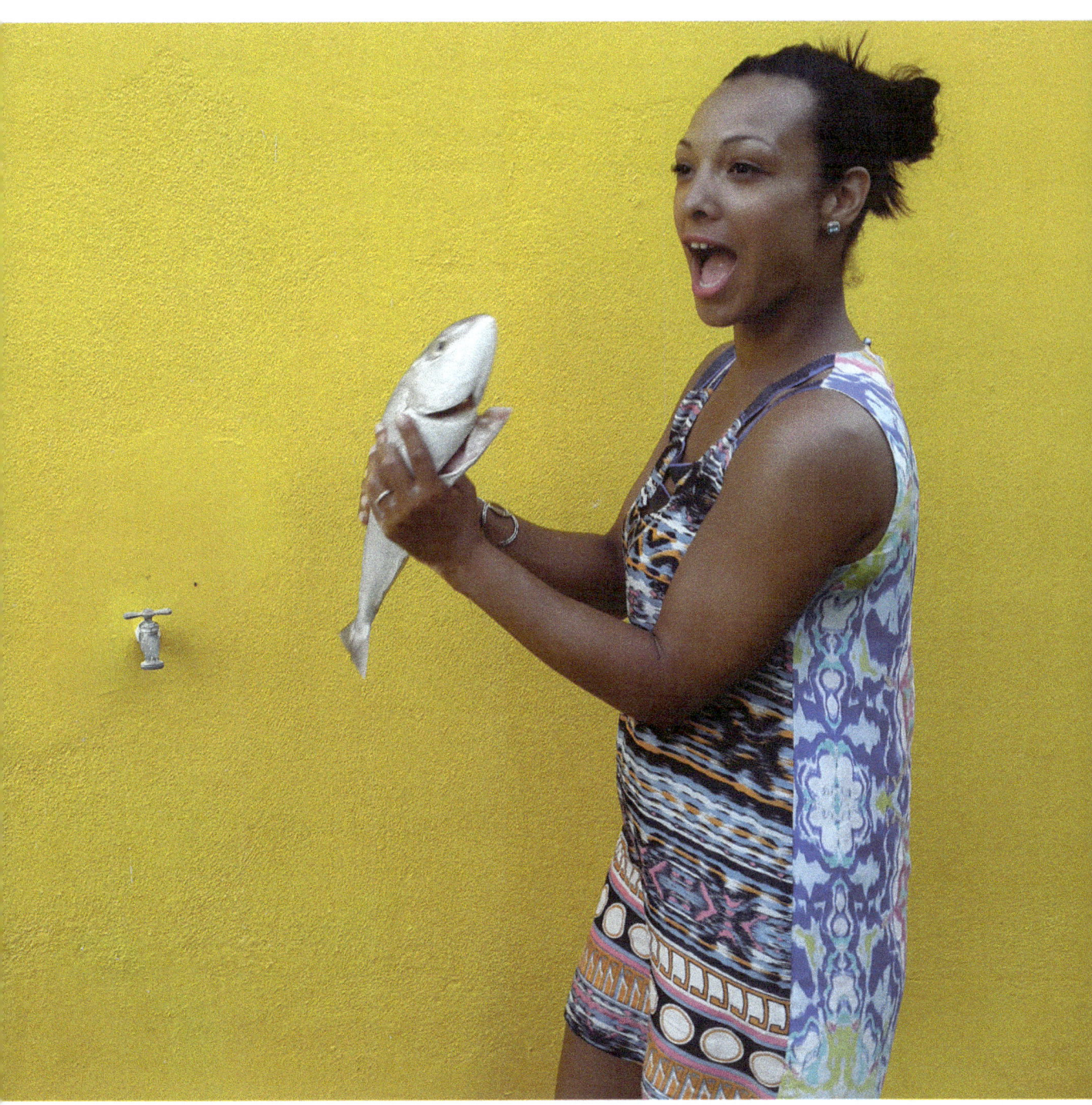

Protein, in the right quantity, is beneficial to your health and seafood can be an excellent source. But what about the fat? Isn't salmon high in fat and doesn't a high fat diet make me gain weight and put me at risk heart disease? The same 100 gram portion of salmon contains between 11 and 13 grams of fat. However, as mentioned in **Healthy (and Downright Essential) Fats and Oils**, we know that not all fats are bad for us. In fact, the right fats can FUEL our bodies and enhance our overall health and wellbeing. And when it comes to seafood, much of the fat is "good fat" that comes from omega-3 fatty acids.

SEAFOOD BENEFITS: OMEGA-3 FATTY ACIDS

Omega-3 Fatty Acids are essential to human health and nutrition. You may have heard about omega 3's before, but what's the big deal? Research has shown that omega-3s can reduce heart disease and stroke, prevent diabetes, moderate cholesterol and even improve the appearance of your skin. They are also a potent, natural anti-inflammatory. Most doctors and nutritionists consider omega-3s essential for overall health and recommend increased quantities in the average North American diet. Unlike proteins, our bodies do not naturally produce essential fatty acids, so we must get them through the food we eat.

Luckily, *the right kinds of seafood* provide an excellent source of omega-3s. Fish, such as wild-caught Pacific or Alaskan salmon, Atlantic/Spanish mackerel, Pacific sardines and herring contain high quantities. The salmon portion mentioned above contains between 1200-1700 milligrams (mg) of omega-3 acids (i.e., fish oil) (USDA, 2017b).

While there are many ways to introduce the benefits of omega-3s into your diet (e.g., some seeds and fish oil supplements), a delicious approach is to simply consume seafood on a regular basis. Even if salmon, or fish in general, isn't your preference, there are many foods from the world's oceans that provide a wealth of health benefits as part of a nutrient-rich, FUELLED diet. For example, bivalves, such as oysters, clams, mussels and scallops are nutrient-dense and contain amazing quantities of omega-3s and other vitamins and minerals. However, while there are many benefits of consuming the *right* seafood as part of our regular diet, not all seafood is created equal. As a general rule of thumb, try to eat seafood that's lower on the food chain, like sardines, mussels and clams. They don't contain as many toxins like PCBs (polychlorinated biphenyls - highly toxic industrial compounds) or mercury, which are more concentrated as you move higher up the food chain to larger fish like tuna (Mercola, p.93-99, 2017). However, there is a lot more to consider in your selection.

THE WORLD IS RAPIDLY RUNNING OUT OF FISH

If you walk past a local fish market, look on the menu at your favourite restaurant or simply visit the seafood section of your local grocery store, the first thought on your mind is probably not: "Wow, the world is rapidly running out of fish!" In fact, you may even think the opposite, given the vast quantities on display in markets and eating establishments the world over.

The truth is that world population growth combined with an increased global appetite for seafood, has led to commercial fishing practices that are steadily depleting the number of fish and quantities of wild seafood worldwide. Compounded with illegal fishing practices and the disastrous effects of "bycatch" (incidental catch of unwanted or unsellable species), the Monterey Bay Aquarium, North America's top resource for sustainable seafood recommendations, has stated that "Ninety percent of the world's fisheries are now fully exploited, over-exploited or have collapsed" (Monterey Bay Aquarium, "Consumers," 2017). Other studies predict the global collapse of all seafood fisheries by 2050 (Stanford University, 2006)! In other words, the volume of fish that we take out of the water is steadily diminishing the number of fish in the water. At this rate, there will be a day when we will run out – if nothing changes.

That's right. For all of the amazing dietary benefits of seafood, many wild fish populations cannot keep up. And once a species is gone, not only does it accelerate the decline of other species, we lose the benefits that the species brought to our bodies and to our overall health. For example, overfishing of wild Atlantic Cod has nearly decimated the species since the 1990s, along with the associated health benefits found in the wild variety.

To address this decline, practices such as fish farming, otherwise known as aquaculture, have exploded worldwide to meet our insatiable appetite for seafood. While aquaculture isn't new (it's been used for over a century), these practices, combined with rampant seafood mislabeling, can easily mislead consumers into buying inferior products; or worse, buying products that are potentially harmful to our health and longevity.

So what can you and I do about this? I mean, I recommend that you incorporate seafood into your daily or weekly fuel but then I tell you that we are running out of fish. The good news is that there is a profound link between the global fight to create sustainable seafood and our overall health. You see, by helping yourself become healthier, you will simultaneously join a global movement to save the world's sea life from extinction. Sound like a fish tale? Here's how.

SEAFOOD SELECTION

If you're concerned about the alarming trend of depleting fisheries worldwide, the best thing that you can do is to simply ask questions. You will see that the same questions that will lead you to purchase the best seafood for your body will also inspire conservation of the ocean.

Sustainable seafood is seafood that's caught or farmed responsibly. According to their website, "The Monterey Bay Aquarium's Seafood Watch program helps consumers and businesses choose seafood that's fished or farmed in ways that support a healthy ocean, now and for future generations." Seafood Watch is globally recognized and supported as an advocate for our oceans, providing consumers, fisherman, farmers and organizations with information to help them more responsibly select, catch and raise seafood in a sustainable and health conscience manner. The consumer guides and information contained on their website are terrific resources that can assist you with seafood selection at your local restaurant, grocery store or fish market.

The team at Seafood Watch has prepared very informative consumer guides in multiple languages to help you in your selection process. They have even created a mobile app that makes this information readily available in the palm of your hand. Since 1999, they have distributed over 57 million guides and had nearly two million downloads of their free mobile app since it was released. Both the guides and the app follow a simple green, yellow and red signage where green means "Best Choice", Yellow means "Good Alternative" and Red means "Avoid." All categories consider the fishery, habitat, management and a host of other factors that affect each species.

Scientists and researchers throughout the world update this information twice-yearly so that you are always making the most informed decisions possible. As such, the lists may change from year to year. I encourage you to download the Seafood Watch app today. You should also visit http://www.seafoodwatch.org for further details on why sustainable seafood matters and to download the latest consumer guides. These guides will help you avoid seafood species and origins that are high in toxins, pollutants or other contaminants that can be a determent your health and wellbeing. They will also help you identify seafood that is high in omega-3s and other nutrients.

Knowledge is power, so what can we do? Seafood Watch states, 'The easiest and most important thing you can do is ask the question: "Do you serve sustainable seafood?"' Even if your local fishmonger, grocery salesperson or restaurant waiter doesn't know the answer (or even looks at you sideways), you will be making a huge impact, while promoting your overall health. Simply asking the question lets the owners and managers who are responsible for seafood sourcing know that you care about what you eat, as well as how it ended up in front of you. Or, if that question makes you feel uncomfortable, then pull out the list of "Best Choice" seafood options in the Seafood Watch consumer guide and ask if the grocery store, restaurant or fishmonger serves or sells any items from that list.

The next question you can ask is whether or not a fish is farmed or wild. What you want more than anything is wild caught, and line caught if possible. Farmed fish like Atlantic salmon is not the best choice because most farms are very unhealthy operations, unless the Monterey Bay Aquarium has reported otherwise, and farmed fish has an inferior nutritional profile. You should then follow this question by asking where the fish is sourced from. So, overall the dialogue sounds like this: "Hi there. Is that salmon wild or farmed? And where is it from? Alaska? British Columbia? The Atlantic Ocean?" The important thing to remember is that the more questions you ask, the more informed you'll be and the larger the impact you can make. As consumers, we can vote with our dollars. You can ask the same questions next time you're at a sushi restaurant, an upscale eatery or at your grocery store.

By connecting human health with ocean health, we can achieve a FUELLED lifestyle that allows our oceans to thrive for generations to come. I encourage you to learn more about sustainable seafood and to enjoy the numerous health benefits that quality seafood can bring to your diet.

Herbs, Fermented Foods & Better Sweeteners

Along with your colourful and vast range of vegetables, plant-based proteins and seafood, try to add in a variety of amazing live or dried herbs such as:

- Garlic
- Ginger
- Parsley
- Mint
- Turmeric
- Basil
- Cayenne
- Rosemary
- Oregano
- Dill
- And many more...

As well, try to incorporate a tiny bit of fermented foods into your day. Just make sure they're pickled with salt and water, not vinegar. Fermented foods are loaded with microflora (good bacteria) that help strengthen your digestive tract, boost immunity and reduce cravings for sweets. Examples include:

- Pickles
- Kimchi – (a staple in Korean cuisine, a traditional side dish made from salted, seasoned and fermented vegetables

- like cabbage)
- Pickled vegetables
- Sauerkraut
- Miso (a traditional Japanese seasoning made by fermenting soybeans with salt and koji and sometimes rice, barley, or other ingredients. It is a is a thick paste-like substance used in many Japanese dishes, including miso soup.)
- Kombucha (a variety of fermented, lightly effervescent sweetened black or green tea drinks)
- Kefir (a tart, fermented milk drink similar to a drinking-style yogurt)

Furthermore, I would recommend using healthier sweeteners to sweeten your foods and drinks such as:

- Raw, unpasteurized honey
- Organic maple syrup
- Monk fruit
- Stevia
- Dates

Great Grains

Whole grains, taken in small portions, are a wonderful source of nutrition because they contain dietary fibre, B complex vitamins and a host of minerals like iron. They have been a staple in the human diet for centuries. They are plant-based and the body absorbs them slowly, providing sustained, high-quality energy throughout the day, while curbing cravings for junky sweets.

When you hear the word "whole grains" you might think of the note on a box of commercially prepared cereal that states: "Made with Whole Grains." This is often far from the truth however. The best way to get whole grains into your diet is to buy them in a way so that you can clearly see that all components of the grain (the bran, the germ, and the endosperm) are intact. Simply put, you are looking for food that has been minimally processed or "refined." For instance, a bag of brown or wild rice is a perfectly great (whole) grain to start incorporating into your meals, versus spaghetti or corn flakes.

And don't for a moment think that this is going to be boring. You might not be aware but there is a vast range of whole grains out there — it's truly astonishing. Depending on where you grew up, you might have never tried iron-rich teff, protein-rich quinoa or antioxidant-rich Forbidden Rice/Black Rice. I assure you, there is a very interesting and tasty world of grains out there waiting to be discovered by you. I would greatly encourage everyone to step outside of the box—*of instant rice paired with a flavour packet or the famous macaroni and cheese (if that's what you're eating now)*—and experiment with some of the great grains from around the world.

I would also recommend sticking to cooking gluten-free grains as gluten is a

"Trouble Maker" in a lot of people's digestive systems (this will be described in detail in **Eliminating the Trouble Makers**). Gluten-free grains include rice (and rice pasta), quinoa, teff, millet, cornmeal, amaranth, oats (be careful to check that the oats were processed in a plant that does not also process wheat, which would mean that there could be a chance of cross contamination), to name a few. Sprouted grains found in Ezekiel or Genesis or Manna bread in the frozen section of your grocery store are also a great option (especially if you enjoy sandwiches) as they tend not to cause an uproar in your system. Sprouting the grains before making the bread breaks up the troublesome proteins and carbohydrates, using enzymes that are produced in the process, thus making the grains easier to digest, and, as a consequence, easier for your body to extract nutrients from. Finally, grains that contain gluten include all wheat products like bread, whole wheat pasta, pastries, barley, couscous, spelt, rye, farro, kamut, and a few more. Those are the ones I would eat as little of as possible, along with all other refined carbohydrates like cookies.

One important note about all grains, however, is that as nutritious as they are, they still affect blood sugar levels. Being mindful of portion sizes for all grains is always a good idea.

On Eating Meat & Dairy

Eating meat is much debated today. There are many arguments against eating meat and there are equally as many for eating meat. So, this one is entirely up to you and your individual preferences. I want you to feel like you have options and to feel like being FUELLED is sustainable for you for the long-term.

I eat meat. My favourites are buffalo, duck, beef, turkey and lamb. I enjoy eating muscle meat, organ meat and bone marrow. I digest meat very well when I eat it at midday, when my digestive system is at its strongest and I'm at my hungriest. I grew up eating raw beef tartar on special occasions, a Polish tradition, and sucking the sweet bone marrow out of larger, cooked bones. My mother's bone broths and chicken and beef soups are incredible. I also think beef liver and onions is absolutely delicious. These days, when I eat meat instead of seafood or plant-based proteins, I keep it to just once a day and it's never the largest portion of whatever is on my plate. The key here is to make the best choices possible when it comes to selecting and eating meat. The largest portion of anything on my plate is always colourful and green vegetables. When I eat meat, I chose organic, grass-fed (if possible), and from as close to home as possible. I never eat pork or processed meat and I avoid conventionally raised meat as much as I can.

Conventionally raised means "standard," non-organic meat, often raised in a factory farm using harmful industrial agriculture practices. It has a regular sticker on it at the grocery store that doesn't say "organic" or "grass fed." Beware of labels like "natural" that tell us nothing at all and mean nothing, and "hormone free" that just aren't good enough and do not meet enough "healthy-meat" criteria. Note also that, unfortunately, most restaurants serve conventionally raised meat. As factory farming and industrial agriculture practices continue to poison the conventional meat supply with hormones, antibiotics, genetically engineered feed etc., create inhumane conditions for animals to live in and disastrous conditions for our environment and the communities adjacent to these farms, I would avoid all conventionally raised meat if you can. Once hailed as a revolution, industrial agriculture is now an outmoded and unsustainable approach to producing animal food. The US lags far behind many European countries in this matter, as Europeans have made steady progress towards improving the quality of life for farmed animals over the past 30 years. Most certainly, I would avoid processed meats, including all deli meats and conventional sausages. They're simply not good for your body. I know they're cheaper, but when it comes to meat: reduce your portion size, eat it less often and buy the best quality meat you can afford. Then fill up on greens and vegetables and good oils alongside of it. That's the way to go.

The real key is to just try to make better choices when it comes to eating meat. You can also completely opt out for periods of time. As a society we eat way too much meat and we could do well to reduce our intake to just once a day or a couple of times a week. The same goes for dairy. Be picky about making sure your dairy is organic and if you can find out if the animals were grass-fed instead of fed on genetically engineered crops, all the better. I hate to tell you, but eating yoghurt nowadays is just not as healthy as the ads make it out to be. And it's not just the absurd amounts of sugar they add to it, but it's the unhealthy animals they're coming from that is a huge concern that poses a threat to your health. If you are looking to consume probiotics, take a good quality supplement or get creative and make your own kefir.

Overall, I would encourage you to consume a diet high in seafood, greens, colourful vegetables, fresh water, starchy vegetables like sweet potatoes, a variety of fruit, berries, herbs and spices, healthy fats and oils, nuts, whole grains, legumes; moderate in organic meat and dairy; very low in pork and processed meat, alcohol, sugar-sweetened foods and beverages, processed foods, other junk, and refined grains like cakes, cookies and cereals. Basically, avoid or greatly reduce the amount of foods you eat from the top of the FUELLED pyramid, which will do the opposite of FUELLING your body, and poison it instead. Eat as many of the foods from the foundation of the pyramid as you can. You can absolutely do this – I know you can – and tailor it to your individual needs, tastes and cultural preferences.

There are no recipes for meat in this book even though I enjoy cooking and eating organic meat. The reason is because you probably already know how to roast, barbeque and sauté meat, so just opt for organic, good quality, sustainably raised meats as often as you can and limit your portion size and frequency to once per day or a few times per week. You know what to do.

Key Supplements

Although it's absolutely crucial that you learn how to get your body's most essential nutrients from healthy foods and liquids instead of supplements, there are some key supplements that can be incredibly effective in helping people achieve maximum wellness day in and day out. Again, supplements are not a substitute for eating nutritious foods and maintaining a balanced diet rich in vitamins, minerals, and phytochemicals, but they can be used a tool to enhance your nutrient intake, especially when it comes to the top 5 I have listed below.

I would highly recommend including the following as part of your daily FUEL:

1. Probiotics – Multi-strain with 25 to 50 billion CFU (Colony-Forming Units)
2. Vitamin D3 – between 1,000 – 5,000 IU (International Units)
3. Good quality fish oil supplement or Udo's Choice Oil 3-6-9 Blend Vegan Non-GMO oil or vegetarian softgel – omega-3 fatty acids EPA and DHA
4. Good quality multivitamin
5. Optional: A good digestive enzyme to take with your food to help break it down if you're finding you're having difficulty digesting foods or you regularly do not take the time to chew adequately

Why these?

1. **Probiotics** support a healthy immune system and a super healthy digestive system. They contain 'good' bacteria and are an indispensable component of optimal digestion, enhancing your body's ability to absorb nutrients from your food while combatting bloating, constipation, heartburn, abdominal pain and other digestive issues. Probiotics also help increase your energy, improve your mood, make your skin glow and they promote healthy joints. Most North Americans don't consume enough probiotics through their diet and their own stores can be depleted

from the consumption of processed foods and environmental factors related to the way food is grown today. A probiotic is one of the key supplements necessary for optimal health and wellness.

2. **Vitamin D3** is a huge multitasker. It supports immune, bone and brain health while also promoting heart health and the health of your muscles, cells and organs like the pancreas, colon and kidneys. Vitamin D3 can improve your skin and help your body maintain a healthy blood sugar balance. It's also a strong anti-inflammatory which benefits the whole body. However, many people are vitamin D deficient, even those living in sunny places. It's very difficult for most people to get sufficient vitamin D from the food they eat alone, or through sun exposure, and, as a result, a vitamin D3 supplement is one of the most important daily supplements to take. Again, a high-quality vitamin D3 supplement not only combats vitamin D deficiency, but also promotes a wide range of healthy bodily functions. You can ask your doctor for a blood test that shows your vitamin D level so you know how much you need to supplement.

3. **Fish oil supplements** are packed with omega-3 Essential Fatty Acids (EFAs) (specifically EPA and DHA) that you *must* get from your diet because your body is unable to produce them on its own. Omega-3s are FUEL for your brain, decrease your risk of heart disease and stroke while also helping diminish symptoms of depression, anxiety, hypertension, ADHD, joint pain and arthritis. In fact, a study published in the *European Journal of Neuroscience* (Pudell *et al.,* 2013) showed that fish oil reversed all anxiety-like and depression-like behavior changes induced in rats. Fish oil also aids in protecting your body from inflammation and preventing chronic diseases. In addition to all of that, these supplements promote a strong immune system, strengthen your skin, hair and nails and boost your body's ability to absorb nutrients. Because your body cannot produce omega-3s on its own, it's imperative that everyone get enough of this Essential Fatty Acid on a regular basis. The health benefits of omega-3s are numerous and far-reaching, making a fish oil supplement a key component of your daily supplement intake. If you are vegan or vegetarian, or for variety, I would highly recommend using Udo's Choice Oil 3-6-9 Blend Vegan Non-GMO oil or vegetarian softgel.

4. **A good multivitamin** can help "fill in the blanks" with your nutrition and diet even if you are a "healthy eater." First of all, it's important that your mutivitamin contains B vitamins, especially vitamin B12, which play a huge role in maintaining your body's energy levels, helping you fight fatigue and giving your body a significant energy boost. B vitamins also promote heart health and a healthy immune system. A good multivitamin will also help break down proteins, fats and carbohydrates. What to look for, in addition to B vitamins, is that a good multivitamin typically contains vitamin D3, vitamin K, vitamin A, magnesium, calcium, vitamin C, iodine, zinc and selenium. Now, not all multivitamins are created equal. Look for a multivitamin made with whole food ingredients and beware of any that contain artificial colors, preservatives, fillers and binders or allergens like dairy, gluten or soy. Now, this may be surprising, but even if you are a "healthy eater," you may still need to "fill in the blanks" in your nutrition with a good quality multivitamin. There are a few reasons for this. Let's start with environmental factors such as soil depletion, which means that a lot of our soils are not as nutrient-rich or biologically diverse as they could be, or used to be, due to overuse or misuse, so the vegetables, fruits and grains that grow on them, even if organic, are not as rich in vitamins and minerals as they could be or used to be. Another reason a "healthy food" might not be as nutrient-dense as it should be is if it travelled a long way to get to you. The longer the amount of time that lapses between when a vegetable or fruit is picked, seafood is caught, seed is harvested, etc., the less nutrient-dense the food will be. It gets less fresh, less ripe, and loses its nutrients over time. Cooking food can also reduce the nutrients in it. Another reason you might not be getting optimal nutrient levels in your diet even if you are a healthy eater is summarized in the phrase "you are NOT what you EAT, you are what you DIGEST." You may be eating very healthy, plant-based, organic foods, but if your digestion is sub-optimal due to conditions like leaky gut, too much stress, or even just not chewing properly, you may not be deriving the optimal amount of nutrients from the healthy foods you are eating. As a result, you should consider taking a good quality multivitamin supplement daily.

5. Finally, if you have difficulty digesting foods, or do not take the time to chew adequately, **a digestive enzyme** (which

EDUCATE

you take with your food or just before eating) might be right for you. Not everyone needs to take a digestive enzyme, but they can be beneficial for people with digestive problems. Digestive enzymes aid in breaking down difficult-to-digest proteins, starches and fats in your food, which then enables your body to absorb more nutrients from them. Enzymes also promote gut health and healing by controlling pathogens and supporting your immune system. Digestive enzymes can be easily overlooked when it comes to preventing disease and improving a variety of bodily health functions so I strongly encourage everyone to research them and consider adding a digestive enzyme to your daily supplement intake if it's right for you.

It Might Seem Hard But...

At this time, it is probably hard to wrap your mind around eating the way I've been describing. It might feel like a huge change from your current day-to-day life.

But, to start, think of this:

You know the saying: You are what you eat? Well don't be FAST, CHEAP or EASY.

Think about that.

If you want to live an outstanding and vibrant life where food FUELs you, you need to remove the junk that's poisoning your cells on a daily basis (for some of you). You will need to re-evaluate some of the staples in your diet.

That means it's time for some discarding. Collect all of the boxes of pre-packaged foods and junk you have in your fridge and in your cupboards and set them in the middle of the kitchen. Look at them. Study them. Then put them either on a very high shelf or, better yet, in the trash bin. Or give them away to someone else. Do not worry about getting rid of "food." Thank the junk as you toss it out for it has served its purpose to you by showing you what you do *not* need (Kondo, 2014).

After removing the bad stuff, you will want to replace it with good stuff. That means stocking your fridge and kitchen cupboards with whole, real, unprocessed, organic, mostly plant-based foods, healthy fats and oils, deep sea fish, nuts, seeds (and nut/seed butters) and legumes, whole grains and organic or sustainably raised animal products. And get a water filter for your house.

The vast amount of foods that fall into the spectrum of plant-based foods is absolutely astonishing. There is so much out there – nature produces an extraordinary amount of FUEL for the human body. Once you start to really *see* the "produce" section of your local grocery store or start really opening your eyes to what is available at the local farmer's market, you will come to realize that living a FUELLED life can be achieved in many, many ways that can be tailored to your own biological and socio-cultural preferences.

Eliminating the Trouble Makers

One of the side benefits of FUELLING your body is that you naturally start to eliminate what I refer to as the "Trouble Makers" – foods that tend to cause problems in your system. Problems that range from allergies, sensitivities and inflammation, to skin rashes, headaches and brain fog (just to name a few). Some health problems related to these "Trouble Makers" can also be quite severe.

The "Trouble Makers" in many people's systems are:

- Gluten
- Dairy
- Processed Sugar
- Soy
- Eggs
- Caffeine
- Alcohol
- Peanuts
- Nightshade vegetables for some people (tomatoes, eggplants and potatoes)

Once out of the system, a lot of people notice a major improvement in their health, wellbeing and vitality. It's very likely that things are going to clear up for you after just 2 weeks free of these irritants.

I know what you're thinking: *Oh my God, that's so restrictive! No pizza, pasta, soda pop, happy hour highballs?* Yes. Getting FUELLED means you stop poisoning or hurting your body and start FUELLING it instead. However, as I always say: There are plenty of foods you are still eating while eliminating all of the above, even if just for 2 weeks, despite the fact that it sounds very strict at first to most people. You can still wholeheartedly enjoy (organic) protein like beef and chicken, a bounty of colourful vegetables, starchy vegetables, grains like rice and quinoa, berries, fruits, all other nuts and their butters, seeds and their butters, all of your greens, herbs, etc. Smoothies can turn into creamy popsicles for dessert and roasted sweet potatoes with rosemary and sea salt curb those salty/sweet snack cravings. And don't worry, in Part 3 *Transform*, I provide a FUELLED Real Food How-To Recipe Guide that shows you how to create remarkable, easy and delicious meals that form the backbone of a healthier, more vibrant you. There are over 100 easy, delicious recipes that will enable you to FUEL your body in the best way and you can enjoy almost every single one of them while eliminating these Trouble Makers.

If you're not totally blown away by how great you feel after two weeks off of these

Trouble Makers then you can reintroduce them one-by-one to see if your system can tolerate them or if any of them starts to cause issues for you again.

The 90/10 Rule for Success

Okay, you've just taken in a lot of information and chances are that you might feel a bit overwhelmed. It is important to know that a healthy person and a healthy way of life includes eating some less healthy foods and drinking some less healthy beverages on occasion – you do not need to stop eating birthday cake on your birthday, a hot fudge ice cream sundae on a sizzling hot summer day, duck poutine when you visit Quebec City, an Art Mel's fish sandwich when you travel to Bermuda, waffles and fried chicken when you visit the Southern USA…And you might still want to enjoy a champagne toast or glass of wine with your loved ones on occasion. No one is trying to take away your special little pleasures, whatever they may be. The key to being FUELLED is to take in maximum nourishment from amazing foods the majority of the time so that your cells are flourishing and you are living a vibrant life, and then go ahead and make some less healthy choices some of the time, like 3-5 days out of a month. But to start gradually, maybe eat something from the not-so-highly recommended foods, like muffins or cake, only once a day and make 90% of everything else you eat plant-based or seafood.

Here's a great way to look at it: Joshua Rosenthal, MScEd, Founder and Director of the Institute of Integrative Nutrition® promotes "eating healthy foods most of the time (90% of the time) and eating less healthy foods on occasion (10% of the time)" (2008). That way, it's easy to follow and easy to FUEL your body!

A great way to start progressing from where you are to where you want to be is to go slowly, with simple replacements. For instance, changing eggs and sausage at breakfast to a smoothie and Ezekiel toast with almond butter. Changing lunch from pizza or pasta to a big bowl of roasted veggies, brown rice and salmon or locally caught fish, and dinner from meat and white potatoes or a cheesy casserole to something lighter and much more nutritious like one of my spinach salads from the *Transform* section of this book topped off with roasted walnuts and hemp seeds. Eating sweet vegetables like carrots, pumpkin, sweet potatoes, beets and onions also curb sweet cravings, so focusing on those is highly recommended when trying to reduce your intake of cakes, brownies, ice cream, candy bars, etc. These vegetables are especially sweet when roasted (see my section **Roasted Vegetables Rock!**).

Keep in mind: FUELLED is not about deprivation. It's not about starvation. It's not about being on a "die-t" where you think you're going to die and you can't imagine how you're going to make it. In fact, it's the total opposite. It's about satisfaction, fulfilment and feeling damn good. It's about boosting your body. You see, when you start eating more real, plant-based foods and good seafood, you will naturally start to "crowd out" other foods you used to eat, meaning that you have no room or appetite for them anymore because you have filled up on the good stuff. As a result, most people see a drastic reduction in hunger pangs and cravings. They already feel full and (physically and emotionally) satisfied.

Food as Medicine

"Let thy food be thy medicine and thy medicine be thy food."

— Hippocrates

I asked you earlier to consider your beliefs around what being "healthy" means to you. Here's one more philosophy that I would like to present to you. It's an oldie but a goodie: The ancient Greek physician Hippocrates (460-377 BC), who is often referred to as the "Father of Modern Medicine" stated: "Let thy food be thy medicine and thy medicine be thy food."

Think about that.

In the Western World, food and medicine are seen as different and separate. However, Hippocrates pointed out that the foods we eat – whether good or bad – impact our overall health and the presence or progression of disease in our body. He wholeheartedly believed in good food and linked the progression of any ailment to poor nutrition and bad eating habits. He taught that the most important principle of medicine was to respect nature's healing forces, which are present inside every living organism. Hippocrates deemed illness to be a natural occurrence that forced people to discover the imbalances in their health. Be good to your body and it will be good to you.

You see, when he advised "Let thy food be thy medicine and thy medicine be thy food" he meant it literally. Good, healthy, whole foods contain so many of the vitamins, minerals, fats, enzymes and nutrients that are essential for keeping our body functioning properly and for warding off disease. Today, scientists are discovering that foods such as fruits, vegetables, grains, beans, and other plants contain synergistic groups of ingredients that provide medicinal benefit – from Resveratrol to Beta-Carotene to Isoflavones – which have aptly been called "phytochemicals," meaning "plant-based" chemicals, as I mentioned earlier in this book. Scientific studies are suggesting that these chemical compounds have an even greater role in human health than we might have previously thought. For instance, Lycopene, part of the carotenoid family, is a pigment that helps give red fruits and vegetables, like beets and tomatoes, their color, and these red pigments in foods are now known to be of benefit in the treatment of cancer.

It bears repeating: "Let thy food be thy medicine and thy medicine be thy food."

The foods you eat and the liquids you drink can help you or they can hurt you. They can heal you or harm you. They can come from a Green Plant or a Cement Plant. You can eat sugar and trans-fat filled boxed cookies or coffee cake for breakfast or you can eat a spinach, avocado and pineapple smoothie with hemp or flaxseeds for breakfast. To overly simplify it and make it funny: You ARE what you EAT so don't be CHEAP, FAST or EASY! Are you eating good food or *food-like products*? Good food has properties (like phytonutrients) that act as helpers and healers in your body — and that good food is the FUEL you need to live a long, healthy, happy life. Study after study has shown that a poor diet = many serious and long-term health problems down the road (or even not so far down the road – like with caffeine ups and downs, alcohol-induced hangovers, gluten-related "foggy brain," or ADHD symptoms). Instead of trying to fix or 'cure' the short or long-term health issues that arise after years of eating poorly, you can take preventative action and use food as your daily medicine for optimal health at *any* stage of your life.

Once you change your thinking from food ≠ medicine, to FOOD = MEDICINE, you will experience a paradigm shift in how you eat and take care of yourself. Think about that - this is one of the most empowering beliefs you can hold in terms of your health that will guide your decisions about food. And the beautiful thing is that when you make the change, your body will be right on board. Once you start to incorporate FUELLED eating principles into your life, your body will thank you. It will shine for you. It knows when you're being good to it and it will be good to you. You will never have to diet again.

Goal Every Day

Every time you eat or drink, it's an opportunity for you to nourish every cell in your body. Consider eating foods that reinforce vital, healthy, strong and magnificent cells. *Raise the Bar* every single day on your expectations of *what food can do for you*. Because it can do a lot more than fill your stomach so that you don't feel hungry.

Modifying your lifestyle is the key to building a strong, lean and resistant body. The daily goal of someone who is totally FUELLED and energized for life is to consume the foods that will help serve their body's functions to the fullest. Foods that will *bring it*! These people are empowered with knowledge, they're totally nourished and have stepped it up to create and sustain an optimal level of well-being. An optimum level of health, energy and vitality they might have thought previously unimaginable.

And they make it fun and simple and fulfilling. A fresh smoothie for breakfast or glass of veggie juice instead of a coffee and muffin or doughnut or boxed cereal with milk. Keeping a fresh salad and an avocado on hand and mixing their own dressing using a healthy oil. Eating walnuts for a snack and carrying a water bottle or coconut water or any other healthy drink they love with them everywhere they go. They opt to *uplevel* their nutrition every single moment they're able to.

Delicious!

Now, my favourite part of all of this is that it can be so delicious. I mean, what's a good life without delicious food? Right?

I read an article in *Vogue* Magazine called "Taking Root" published in October 2015 (US edition) that really speaks to the delicious-ness of eating plant-based foods. In it, the author dives into what he describes as the "current chef-driven, plant centric gastronomic boom" (i.e. the boom in plant-based foods like vegetables, grains, beans, nuts and fruits, being served up in restaurants) that's sweeping over many parts of the world today. He focuses on New York City and presents some of the scientific, nutritional and ethical data behind this wave of change, this shift in the balance of our diet to more real, fresh plant-based foods. Then, he writes, and this is my favourite quote:

"Of course, the data have been accumulating for a long time. What is different now is chefs themselves, who seem, in silent collective assent, to have decided to advance the argument for plants in the eternally more convincing language of pleasure. And have begun sculpting a culinary landscape anew."

The *"language of pleasure."*

I repeat: *Pleasure.*

Yes, the best part of it all is that FUELLING your body is an absolutely delicious undertaking. It's also about abundance. It's about variety. It's about satisfaction. It's about gorgeous aromas drifting out of the kitchen and happy taste buds. This is not about deprivation. It's not about starvation. It's not about being on a "die-t." In fact, when you start eating more real, plant-based foods and good seafood, you will naturally start to "crowd out" other foods because you have filled up on the good stuff. As a result, most people see a drastic reduction in hunger pangs and cravings. They already feel full and (physically and emotionally) satisfied.

The great thing is that you don't even have to go far to experience this new culinary landscape, or spend loads of money. You can do it yourself at home in your kitchen and your local farmer's markets and grocery and health food stores provide all the best ingredients you will ever need.

When you are ready to try this on and are ready for a transformation and you buy some great real foods, but experience anxiety, overwhelm, confusion or get just downright stumped when you get home and get into the kitchen…and you don't know what to cook or where to start, I have thought of you. In Part 2: *Inspire*, I help you overcome all of those emotional obstacles and in Part 3: *Transform*, I provide a FUELLED Real Food Recipe How-To Guide that is in line with the teachings in this part of this book. The recipes demonstrate that healthy, life giving, nourishing foods are surprisingly easy to prepare and absolutely delicious to eat. And, going back to the article, what is more convincing than *pleasure*?

Lifestyle Recommendations

"Doing the best at this moment puts you in the best place for the next moment."
— Oprah Winfrey

Really being able to *bring it* every single day comes from living a life where you are enhancing your human potential day in and day out, or as often as you can. Getting FUELLED and optimizing your cell functioning through the foods you eat has been the focus and scope of this book but I would be doing you a disservice to leave out a brief section on lifestyle recommendations, which, epigenetics teaches us, also affect your cellular health and how your genes behave.

Once you start to eat healthier and really FUEL your body, it becomes easier to make lifestyle choices that enable you to increase your productivity, decrease your stress and anxiety, boost your mood, shed excess weight and motivate yourself to achieve your dreams. Lifestyle changes are an essential component to feeling more energized and passionate about life.

- **Strive for 8 hours of solid sleep every night** — It's best to sleep from 10 p.m. to 6 a.m., as the most regenerative sleep often occurs between 10 p.m. and 2 a.m. That means you are horizontal at 9:30 pm. Sleep benefits your heart, your mind, and your body. Not getting enough can be very bad for your health. If you struggle with anxiety or insomnia, please learn what you can about overcoming these health challenges and get as much support as you can so that you can sleep as soundly as possible. I struggled with a crippling insomnia for half a year, so I can relate to you if that is what you are going through. It was absolutely horrible. I was a shadow of my former self. But I fully recovered without the use of prescription drugs and made some necessary changes to my life and environment to ensure I stayed healthy afterwards. Being a great sleeper will help you THRIVE and keep your DRIVE ALIVE!

- **Exercise or do a form of physical activity every day** — Working out and getting yourself moving and breathing is an incredible energy booster, so challenge yourself to add more physical activity into your regular routine. The body enjoys both high-impact workouts that increase your heart rate and get your blood pumping, as well as low-impact practices like yoga, breath work and other, less-intense forms of exercise, like rebounding on a mini-trampoline, which can make you feel rejuvenated and energized afterwards. Be sure to find things you love to do or find a way to love what you wish you were doing by incorporating music, picking a great location, enlisting a friend, joining a class, getting an accountability buddy or health coach, or tracking your progress on social media for extra support and that fun social element. If you don't know where to start, start with taking the stairs everywhere you go and park further away from the entrance to your workplace, grocery store, etc., and walk the extra distance every chance you can. Try as best as you can to not sit down for long periods of time.

- **Eat mindfully** — One of the easiest ways to start changing your eating habits is to become more aware of your eating. Sit down at the table when you eat and take the time to truly enjoy your meal. Don't eat in front of the TV or computer or distract yourself during meals by constantly checking your phone or reading the news. I would encourage you to set an intention before eating or to say a prayer. This doesn't have to be complicated and can be as simple as: "I am so grateful for this delicious food. May it nourish me and make me stronger." As well, I would recommend making lunch your largest meal, at midday, a time that you really need to FUEL yourself for the whole day ahead and when your digestion is at its peak functioning level. The fact that dinner is the largest meal for most people confuses me greatly as it is the last meal of the day, right before they go to sleep. You needed that FUEL earlier in the day to support all your brain and bodily activity. Don't be afraid to be a little different and eat less at night and much more during the daylight hours.

- **Breathe deeply** – Deep breathing is the first thing we forget to do when we get to the office, start to read the flood of email that has come in and begin to stress over our workload. But it's really the first thing we should do and funnily enough, it's something our society has to re-learn to do. Deep breathing means breathing from your belly, using your diaphragm. There are many resources available to assist you with the "How To" aspect of this, so find a video, book, quote, handout, podcast, or whatever works for you and start to learn to breathe. The benefits are truly incredible. Deep breathing makes you calmer, happier, reduces stress, brings clarity, stimulates the lymphatic system, detoxifies the body, relieves pain and releases tension, massages your organs, supplies oxygen to the muscles, improves the quality of your blood, increases digestion, improves your nervous system function, strengthens the lungs and heart, assists in weight control and boosts energy levels. Need I say more?

- **Learn to love yourself** – Psychologist Gay Hendricks often states that learning to love yourself is *the* key mindset that can help you end the cycle of negative thoughts, toxic eating patterns, and chronic dissatisfaction (2011). It also will provide an incredibly solid foundation for releasing unwanted weight. And I fully agree. It doesn't matter if you're a man or a woman, if you want to take your transformation to another level then you must learn the most powerful tool you can use to feel happy and fulfilled in every area of your life – and that is radical self acceptance and true self love. Because when you learn to truly love yourself - just as you are – Guy Hendricks teaches, your body often has a way of becoming what you've wanted it to be.

- **Expand your 'Circle of Genius'** — Motivational speaker Jim Rohn famously said that "You are the average of the five people you spend the most time with." As a part of creating a magnificent life, you need to take steps to surround yourself with people who inspire you, support you, motivate you and lift you up to the next level. Find friends who are living at a higher level, and seek out wisdom teachers — even famous ones like Tony Robbins, Albert Einstein, Deepak Chopra, Joel Osteen, Oprah Winfrey or Trent Shelton — who will enlighten you and show you new pathways for overcoming obstacles and achieving your dreams.

- **Boost your brain power** – Engage in fulfilling work. Develop your spirituality. Take on an Attitude of Gratitude. Practice forgiveness. Try a new hobby. Learn a new skill. Take on a practice of daily expansion (either emotional, intellectual, spiritual). Take in enlightening podcasts, movies, audiobooks, books and other forms of information. Learn how your brain can be taught to reach far beyond its present limitations and then practice what you learn.

- **Become financially smart** — Do what it takes to get motivated about becoming financially smart and successful. Do your best to earn the most you can with your skills and talents, spend wisely, do not accumulate bad debt, save as much as you are able to, learn about investing to see if it's right for you (in real estate, stocks, bonds, whatever works for you). Emotional eating can be tied to factors in your life that stress you out, put you in a mindset of scarcity, make you feel like you are lacking, so you want to be proactive about keeping yourself strong and solid insofar as money is concerned.

- **Educate yourself on hair, makeup and skincare products**: Be careful of what you use on your body. Some products contain harmful chemicals that have been linked to cancer and other health problems. Our skin absorbs what we put on it so do your research before you buy so that you know which ingredients to avoid.

- **Discover your life purpose** – Make it your business to know what your gifts are and then to uncover and pursue your mission in life. There is an incredible lifeforce that comes from living on-purpose, for something that is larger than yourself.

- **Beware the 4 D's** (from a spiritual teacher of mine): **Distractions, Detractors, Desires and Detours** — A lot can be said about all of these but basically they speak to the following: Beware Distractions and, instead, stay present in your life, in your career, with your family, with your friends and with yourself because every day is precious and you want to "be there" for it; Beware Detractors, those who take away your energy and make you feel less than your best – make sure you are surrounded by people with whom you have healthy, happy relationships; Beware Desires, i.e. your motives, and check in on them every so often to make sure they are good and in alignment with your higher purpose; and Beware Detours, be sure to stay on course with your personal mission and purpose in the world (Peets, p.67-68, 2015).

- And, as an added bonus, try to enjoy as many as you can of what I call **my 6 S's**, especially if stress shows up a lot in your life —

1. Sound **Sleep,**
2. **Spa**-time (or massages and touch, aromas and restorative practices in any healthy form at any location that works for you),
3. Safe and Seductive **Sex**,
4. **Superfoods,**
5. Satisfying **Sports** (running, swimming, walking in nature, skiing, weight lifting, soccer, whatever you can fall in love with), and

6. **Spirituality** (whatever that means to you).

I will leave these healthy pleasures for you to incorporate any way you would like to in your life.

Body Stronger to Serve the World Longer

"The secret of change is to focus all of your energy, not on fighting the old, but on building the new."

— Dan Millman, Way of The Peaceful Warrior

Many of us want to improve our health so that we have the energy to pursue our passions and live our lives to the fullest. It's nearly impossible to achieve your dreams without having the physical and mental stamina to do so. A big part of living a magnificent life is having the energy to do what makes you happy.

Consider the following:

- What gives you energy and excites you?
- What are your dreams?
- What are your goals?
- What do you desire in all the different areas of your life?
- What gifts were you brought on the earth to leave as your legacy and to share with others?
- What is your personal mission in life?
- With revitalized energy, a stronger and healthier body, a clearer mind, and cells functioning at their optimal level, can those dreams come true?

You see, my belief is that we were all brought on this earth for something much bigger than ourselves. My passion is helping people gain their energy edge and close the gap between where they are and where they want to be though FUELLING their body so that it works at an optimal level. I love helping people achieve a vibrant and fulfilling life that they might have thought previously unimaginable for themselves, using integrative nutrition techniques and the principle of true **FUEL – Food Unleashing Energy for Life**, and then seeing them succeed in the progressive realization of worthy goals and dreams after that. Because having a personal mission is so important but having the energy to realize your personal mission and create your dreams really matters at the practical day-to-day level.

I get excited when I think of a new way to explain the philosophy of *Raising the Bar* on what food can do for you (in terms of your optimal wellbeing) and when I think about how implementing this mindset can help take your already successful life to the *next level*. I value the power of education

+ inspiration + coaching in the true transformation of people's lives. I am driven by the challenge found in how to get people to tackle and conquer the optimal health/nutrition/food piece in their lives that they either ignored so far, feared, or thought was too difficult to grasp or to integrate so far. My mission is to help you succeed in that arena and then see you move towards the progressive realization of all your worthy goals and dreams after that.

Because health is not a goal, it is a launchpad. Because achieving optimal health is *the* best springboard for achieving all of your biggest dreams. It is a vehicle, not a destination.

What do you want to be healthy for?

Whatever it is, I would love to see you totally FUELLED and ready to power through anything because you are unstoppable!

"Go forth and set the world on fire," St. Ignatius of Loyola urged every one of us.

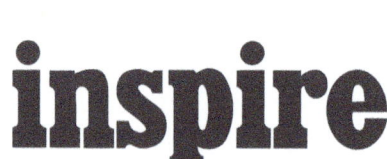

Every step in the next section has the power to change your personal reality.

It is time for some inspiration.

In Part 1: *Educate* you learned some of the practical fundamentals about nutrition, how food impacts the cells, and your body's vital needs. You now know which foods, nutrients and supplements FUEL the body for maximum health benefits. Pretty cool, right? I mean, you now have the knowledge to understand how real food provides the best FUEL for life, and, consequently, you now have the knowledge to understand how to unlock the potential of **FUEL = Food Unleashing Energy for Life**.

Talk about an overhaul of your health and wellness mindset. Talk about empowering. Talk about life changing.

Or is it?

To take your knowledge and start on a new path without considering what's in front of you could leave you with broccoli, eggplant and garlic that are stashed at the very back of the fridge and turning brown two weeks after reading this book. You set out to try a new way of eating and then got bored or stressed or uncertain and gave up, yet again. Enter disappointment, negativity and that downhearted-in-your-soul-way-of-being associated with the feeling of failure that comes from a perceived lack of progress or accomplishment.

Knowledge Is Power? No, knowledge is only potential power.

You see, it has been said that the results you're getting in *any* area of your life are a reflection of what you're really *committed* to. Notice that that means the results you're getting in any area of your life are *not* a reflection of what you *know*, or understand to be true.

Napoleon Hill said "Knowledge is only potential power. It becomes power only when, and if, it is organized into definite plans of action, and directed to a definite end (1937)."

Loosely translated, that means you need to set some goals and get an action plan.

In fact, not only do you need to set some goals and get an action plan, but, if you really want to feel empowered, you need to set yourself up for success in a *big* way.

It's time to get *committed* to getting FUELLED.

It's time to get inspired, excited, enthusiastic and confident. It's time to get your heart and soul switched on to your new outlook.

This section will help you close the gap emotionally between where you are now and where you want to be. It will help you overcome the mental and emotional blocks and hurdles that stand in the way of you becoming a healthier you – like your fear of leaving your comfort zone. It will help you establish your "Why" so that you can clearly articulate your reasons for wanting to get FUELLED for LIFE. And then it will support you as you tap into the awesome power of visualization to create a vision of success as relates to your living a healthy, happy and energized life.

Passion is a key ingredient in your success, so pay attention to this section.

I wish you all the success in the world as you embark on this journey of achieving optimal health and creating an abundant, passionate and FUELLED life!

Overcoming Fear

The great paralyzer in any mission is fear. Fear shows up in our lives as:

- Fear of change
- Fear of what it might cost
- Fear of failure, and, everyone's favourite
- Fear of leaving your comfort zone

When we allow fear to gain a foothold, we will be paralyzed. We will get stuck. We will quite possibly go right back to our old habits and old mindset. We might not hit our goal. We might not be faithful to our dream.

You know how it is.

You set a goal – Today is your day. You have just read/listened to/seen/heard something that really moved you. A new and awesome idea. An immensely empowering perspective. Something you struggle with that has been simplified and made more approachable. Your

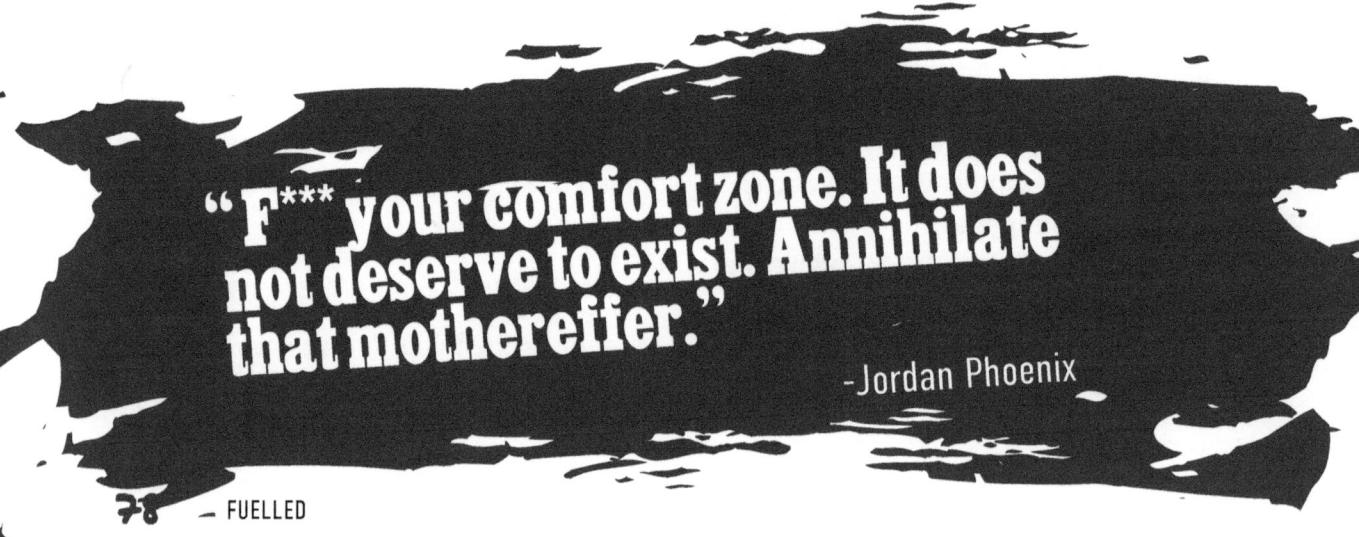

"F*** your comfort zone. It does not deserve to exist. Annihilate that mothereffer."
–Jordan Phoenix

mind is overflowing with dreams and desire. Your heart throbbing as you feel a greater life purpose, a greater sense of self, a zest for life rekindled. Your mission is clear and you are committed to succeed. You tell yourself that this time, yes, finally this time, I will make that change and reach that goal. You are unstoppable.

But do you continue to dance even after the music has stopped? Did you capture those goals and the vision that you had when you were motivated *in that moment*? A vision of a future you that's vibrant, healthy and driven to make the most of each day that you're given. Or did you falter when the emotional high wore off, left longing for change and unsure of your path? You remind yourself how many times you've tried before, only to result in perceived failure of accomplishment.

Goals can be both an inspiration and they can cause us to run and hide from fear of the unknown. They can motivate us to strive for a better life, push us to accomplish more than we ever thought possible and inspire us to positively impact the lives of others. But substantive goals also carry with them the challenges of discipline, perseverance and dedication. You must face these challenges, as well as emotions like uncertainty, overwhelm and fear when they come your way. Some days, you look left, you look right, and you wonder where your enthusiasm slipped off to. Some days you find you have to pick yourself up and push yourself forward towards the achievement of the goals that you set. And for some people there are those days where that push may appear futile when confronted with the obstacles and fears that are a natural part of doing something amazing that would fulfill your soul but is outside of your comfort zone.

When we step into uncharted territory, especially in the beginning, we are confronted with the ever-present choice to overcome obstacles like change, uncertainty and fear and advance ourselves forward, ever closer to our goals, our vision; or to simply give up and call it quits when the going gets tough. This choice is sometimes made harder when we can't see the fruit that is slowly growing from the seeds that we have planted. We are a culture that wants results ASAP.

Taking the first step of our journey can be incredibly exciting, however, the hardest part is often found somewhere along the path between that pivotal first step and our final destination.

So you must ask yourself these questions:

- What will help me stay the course and reach my goal?
- Do I have a strategy or an action plan?
- How can I avoid the paralysis that occurs from the negativity, guilt, disappointment or shame associated with that feeling of failure when it comes, because of one day, two days or a week off course?

Make no mistake about it, emotions play a role in whether or not we successfully achieve

> "If you can't fly then run, if you can't run then walk, if you can't walk then crawl, but whatever you do you have to keep moving forward."
>
> —Martin Luther King, Jr.

our ultimate dreams. Empowering or positive emotions like *interest, joy, hope, gratitude, cheerfulness, serenity, inspiration, confidence, enthusiasm, satisfaction, enjoyment, love, awe* and *fuelled* keep us on course and ever moving forward towards the realization of our ultimate dreams. This is helpful consciousness. However, disempowering or negative emotions like *fear, indifference, frustration, overwhelm, boredom, dread, anxiety, envy, stress, worry, discontent, disappointment* and *guilt* can lead us to stagnate. And don't all of these disempowering emotions really boil down to fear at their core?

These emotions can impact the vision we set out for ourselves, for better or for worse.

So I'm here to tell you that you do not want to stand in your own way. You do not want to be the biggest obstacle in the achievement of your own personal success. You do not want your disempowering emotions, like fear of change, cost, failure and of venturing outside of your comfort zone, to stand in the way between who you are and who you want to become.

And that's exactly why this section exists between *Educate* and *Transform*. Between the information in the text and the FUELLED Real Food How-To Recipe Guide. Because knowledge isn't power. It's *potential* power. Information alone is rarely what motivates people to uplevel their health and their lifestyle. It's necessary that we feel *inspired* to make different choices, adopt better eating habits and envision a new future for ourselves.

I am going to help you switch on, mobilize, trigger, call up, harness — whatever word you want to use —all the positive and empowering emotions you can about your journey towards FUELLING your body in the best way — and getting FUELLED for the next phase of your life!

First, I am going to walk you through my simple, no frills, 3 Step Process to overcoming fear:

Step 1: Feel the fear. Wow, that's scary. *I am going to quit eating processed sugar and the holidays are around the corner.* Great job. Then notice that it's all in your head. It's invisible. I know its power can seem immense and real, but it doesn't physically exist. In fact, if you were a different person with a different experience of life and a different outlook, this fear might not even have come to surface in your thoughts and emotions. It does not have to exist.

Step 2: Feel the fear and do it anyway. Push it aside. Think: *This is for my higher good. For the person I want to become.* Take whatever you're afraid of doing or being and chunk it down. Break it down into small steps that are less intimidating. Maybe steps that you could tackle in a day. *I will substitute all processed sugar with raw honey.* And if one of those steps scares you, make that step even smaller. *I will go to the store today at 5pm and buy raw, unpasteurized honey.* Make it as small as you want and then say "Get lost, Comfort Zone, I'm trying new things," and push, encourage or bribe yourself to do it. Whatever it takes. Just take one of those small steps and conquer it. Just move forward every single day. You will feel your confidence go up, your sense of hope increase, and you might even feel like a different person.

Step 3: Discover the Awesome Power of Visualization. AKA Get a vision for yourself. Through visualization, we direct

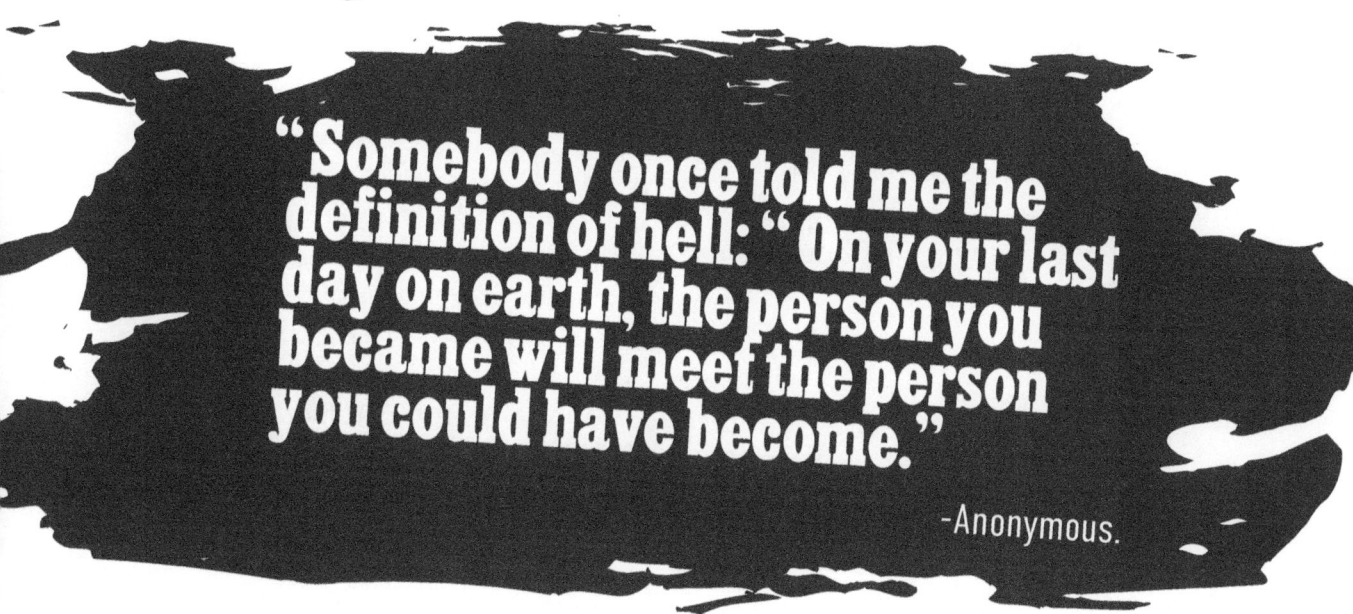

"Somebody once told me the definition of hell: "On your last day on earth, the person you became will meet the person you could have become."

-Anonymous.

> "Before you start, visualize your destination"
>
> -Marie Kondo

The Awesome Power of Visualization

our mind and we become the master of our emotions. We set ourselves up for success in a BIG way. By seeing ourselves as already successful at our goal, before we even start, we positively impact our emotions in an intense way, and increase our rate of success immensely. This works even more powerfully when you tie in "I AM" statements (Osteen, 2012) where you declare yourself as already having all the qualities you dream of having, even if you don't have them quite yet: "I AM A LEAN, MEAN, ENERGY MACHINE!!!" And if we revisit our vision often, when we close our eyes and tap back into our dream, then at those times when the journey becomes arduous, when we are tempted to quit, we regain hope. We get re-**FUELLED**.

The purpose of visualization is to close the gap emotionally between where you are now and where you want to be. You see, it's absolutely necessary to paint a vivid picture in your mind of what your life will be like and how you will feel once you accomplish any goal that you have set. This imagery contains the power to push you towards the realization of those goals and to boost you up even when you encounter obstacles or setbacks along your journey.

To do this, you must look at your goal and continually ask yourself, "Why?"

Why did you seek out and buy this book? What is it about **FUELLED** that caught your eye? What are you hoping to achieve by reading this book? Why do you desire to become healthier or to change your outlook and lifestyle for the better? As Tony Robbins often asks, "What's your Why?"

You are far more likely to complete your journey or reach the goal that you have set for yourself if you can clearly articulate your reasons for wanting to achieve it.

Think about it: Do you dream of a future you, a more vibrant and healthy "You" that you have never known? Remember, health is not a goal – it's a launch pad. If you stick to it, you will find that getting FUELLED can be the catalyst that propels you to excel in so many other areas of your life. When you have the energy, when you have the vitality, when you have optimal health, your life is propelled forward and made better in all aspects.

Your visualization, your "Why?", has to be rock solid. Just as the foundation for skyscrapers is drilled deep into the bedrock, your vision, your purpose for achieving the goals that you have set must also be deep-rooted in your very being. You must drill down into your soul to lay an unshakable foundation that cannot be moved or cracked when you're faced with obstacles, detours, detractors, distractions or desires. Come on, you know it: temptation, social pressure, holidays, break ups, family crises, home renovations, work potlucks, job stress, job travel, loneliness, anxiety, boredom, exhaustion, bad days, bad habits, and you name it *what else can go wrong* will show up on your path to success. You absolutely have to find the "Why?" that inspires and drives you, at any cost and at any moment, during those trying times. You have to visualize the real you, a healthier you, the one with a new outlook on health and powerful goals for the future, living out the benefits and joys that are only found through the accomplishment of the goals that you have set. How exciting is that?! You then have to harness that inspiration to move forward. You have to review and renew your intentions to recharge your mission. Remember, true success is the progressive realization of worthy goals. To reach them, you need clarity. You need a vision.

That is why I've included this section on inspiration and visualization in between the *Educate* and *Transform* sections of this book. A critical component of your journey is to *Inspire* yourself. And I really want you to succeed. If you do not spend time developing a picture in your mind of why you want this and what you're going to get out of it, then the chances of rebounding or quitting greatly increases. And if you, like I, truly value health, then you wouldn't want to rebound or quit.

So, once you nourish your body and are FUELLED and THRIVING, what are you going to do? What do you see yourself doing? Being? Feeling?

Go beyond the generic: "I want to feel more energized," or, "I want to shed this excess weight to feel better" to something more vivid and empowering, like:

- "I want to wake up every morning and feel healthy, vibrant, and ALIVE. I want to use my boundless energy to conquer the day, to realize my dreams, and to take the holidays and adventures I've always longed for, like making the trek see the ancient ruins of Machu Picchu in Peru or white water rafting in the Grand Canyon. I want to fall asleep every night SMILING and totally SATISFIED with my day."

- Or "With increased confidence in my body and in my ability to stick to and conquer my goals, along with the happiness and attractiveness that's overflowing in my life from unlocking the true potential of **FUEL = Food Unleashing Energy for Life**, I want to finally meet that amazing person I know is out there for me so that I can experience the love and passion and intimacy I know I deserve and have always dreamed of, but was always afraid of going after. I can't wait to meet this person and show them who I am and how much I can love them!"

- Or "I want to have the energy, stamina and vigor to provide for my family, those I love most in the world, those who are the dearest to me, and to live a long, healthy life so that I can see many generations of my family grow up. I want to stop the cycle of sickness and disease that came before me in my family and so I want to be a strong role model for my kids and their kids to look up to, and to help them and encourage them to realize their dreams and to become healthy – become **FUELLED** – for a better life."

I encourage you to paint your story and visualize your goals as vividly as you possibly can. You must become intimately connected to your goal and feel your passion towards it burning like a bonfire in your soul. I want you to succeed, and visualization is a key component of your success.

And here's the thing: It won't always be about checking in with your vision to keep yourself on course with your mission. Studies show that if you consistently do something for six months of your life then you are far more likely to do it for the rest of your life. It becomes who you are – who you see yourself as *being*. You identify with it: *this is the way I eat, the way I do life*. Would you trade six months of perseverance for a lifetime of payback? Sounds like a good trade-off to me! So, let's spend some time developing your vision and your purpose for why you want to live a **FUELLED**, energized and outstanding life.

I would encourage everyone to embrace the power of visualization and to practice flooding yourself with emotions and feelings that empower you about your future. Below, I provide an example visualization that you may use to help start your journey, but you have to finish it with your own personal goals and dreams. It's an adaptation of one I heard in Fiji that inspired me, written by a real

Energy Rocket herself, Margaret 'Chili' Irving. I wish you all the success in the world as you embark on this journey of achieving optimal health and creating an abundant, passionate and **FUELLED** life!

And remember:

"Don't let others tell you what you can't do. Don't let the limitations of others limit your vision. If you can remove your self-doubt and believe in yourself, you can achieve what you never thought possible."

— Roy T. Bennett, The Light in the Heart

Example Visualization

Start One Day

So you start one day. They say there's no time like the present. TODAY is your day.

You're sick and tired of being sick and tired. You make a decision to lay your FOUNDATION and achieve cellular fitness. You are committed to *Raising the Bar* on what food can do for you and to putting the wheels in motion to begin **FUELLING** your body. You look at yourself in the mirror and envision yourself a lean, mean, energy machine. People can feel your presence when you walk in a room. You have so much energy and vitality and are excited about creating your life's dreams.

Eating to Energize

You start eating to energize and it opens you up to a whole new world were food **FUELS** you. Where every time you eat, it's an opportunity to nourish your body to its cellular core. At first, it's not a great effort. You start eating FRESH, REAL FOOD. And it doesn't have to be super fancy or complicated. Just simple ingredients, prepared simply.

Eating this way leaves you feeling full so you start to cut out boxed and packaged foods and replace them with real food that you prepared that doesn't have an ingredients list on the side of it. You could never decipher those lists anyway. You even stop drinking sodas and coffee. This becomes so easy when you replace them with alternatives like coconut water, green juices, delicious smoothies, fresh water, and iced peppermint tea made with unpasteurized honey. You are eliminating toxins from your body and getting AMPED on life. Step after Step, Day after Day, You start to feel Results. The morning and afternoon sugar and caffeine cravings that you WERE A SLAVE TO disappear, and you awaken refreshed. And...happy.

You are in control of how you **FUEL** your body.

Gaining Momentum

You decide to try out essential fats & oils and you find them delicious. You wonder why you ever carried guilt about eating fat and oils. You notice your skin starts to clear up and GLOW.

Inches start to shed from your waistline and you maintain your momentum for at least six months, because research shows that if you do anything for six months, there is an 80% chance you will do it for the rest of your life.

Taking on the Heart of a Champion

Your body starts to change. And you start to push yourself, adding more and more *Super* – natural – *foods* into your breakfast, lunch and dinner. Replacing old habits with new ones that propel you ever forward. And each push is really a metaphor for who you are becoming as a person. **You are starting to take on the heart of a Champion** – knowing and feeling that each step is taking you closer to your best self.

And it starts to impact your entire Psychology. You are committed. You stay the course, even when the going gets tough. You feel STRONG. You know your goals and you visualize your future self. You mentally push aside anyone who holds you back. You love them, but you don't let others tell you what you can't do. This is your life. **You are a Champion.**

You start to incorporate exercise into your daily morning routine. You change your biochemistry so that your life isn't flat anymore. All of a sudden you are feeling a natural physical high. And you're powering through resistance and creating a compelling future for yourself. Because that's really what the transformative power of nutritional energy – of getting **FUELLED** – is all about. It's about *Food Unleashing Energy for Life*. It's about **FUELLING** your cells so that you can create and sustain a level of energy, health and vitality that you use to create a magnificent life. It's about claiming your nutritional advantage. You are gaining your Energy Edge.

And as you push through any resistance, you condition your mind and WILL POWER too. Each step, each trial, each challenge more deeply aligning you with your purpose. And remember, your brain always remembers, whether it be with physical OR emotional training.

Victory Becomes Your Identity

And then what happens is Physical and Emotional Mastery become your identity. They become the driving forces that carry you for the rest of your life. And you then have the ability to turn on the Energy whenever you need it. In those trying moments. In those moments when you have to totally step up and step into any obstacle that you might have and power right through it, knowing that YOU are always able to access that Energy Edge and that HEART of a Champion you tapped into within yourself.

Food Unleashes Energy for Life

And it all started because you made a FIST POUNDING decision to take action. To make a difference in your Life by making a change that, in fact, transforms your entire life. And so, not only will you be able to go after your own dreams, you will be able to share your gifts, knowledge and passion with others... things that you were brought on the Earth to leave as your legacy. Because my belief is that we were brought on this Earth for something much bigger than ourselves. With a renewed outlook, revitalized energy and powerful goals for your future, your dreams really can come true.

Totally Fuelled

Like a True Warrior, you are in a state of grace, TOTALLY FUELLED and ready to power through anything because YOU are unstoppable!!!!

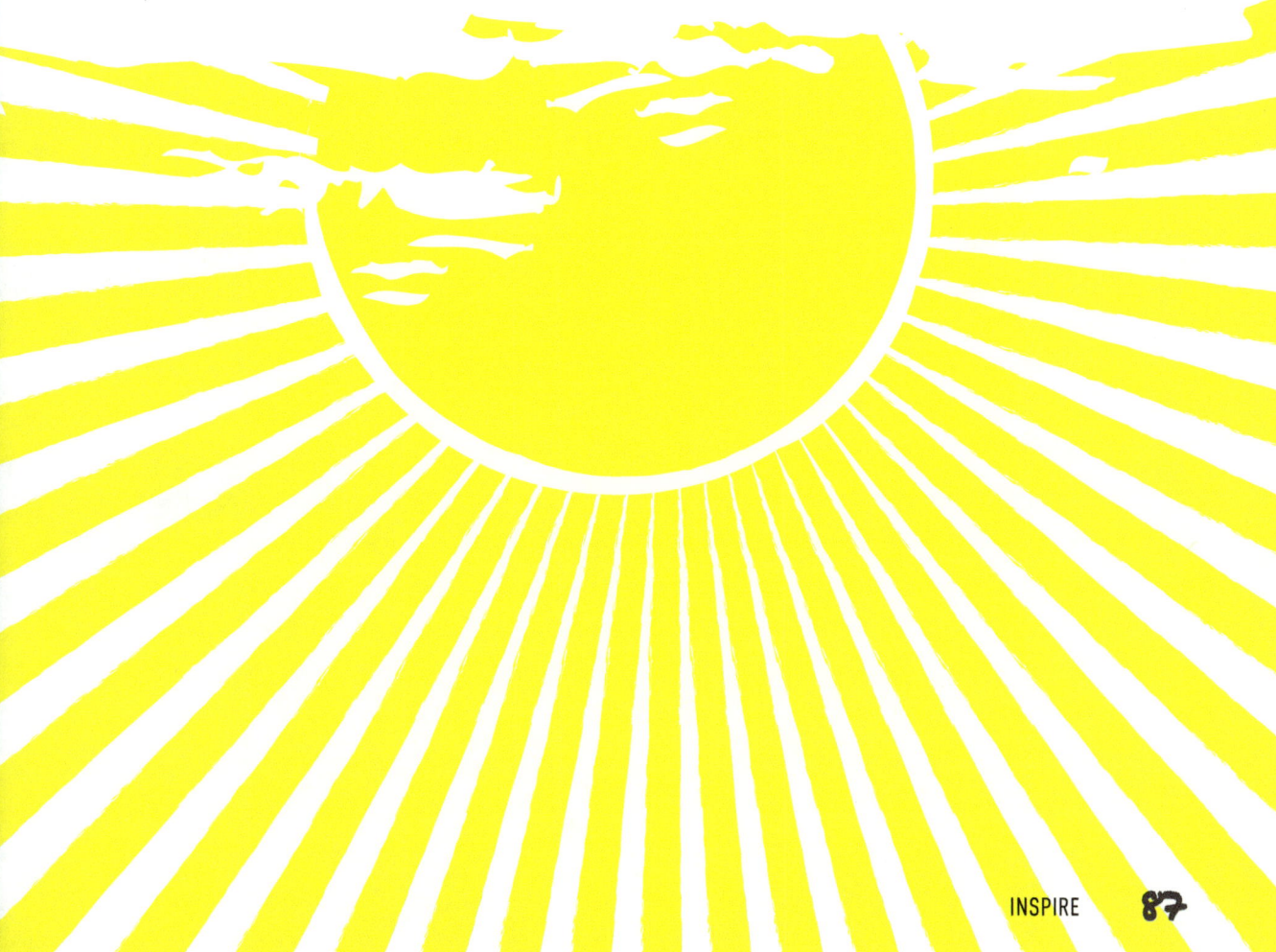

transform

FUELLED

Let's Do This.

It's time to apply all the knowledge contained in the *Educate* section and all of the passion gained from the *Inspire* section of this book to FUEL your cells and propel yourself forward.

This section shows you *how* to transform your life, starting with the basics. It is your FUELLED Real Food How-To Recipe Guide. There are over 100 easy, delicious recipes that will enable you to nourish your body in the best way — and get FUELLED for the next phase of your life!

Before you start, two words of advice.

1: Deepak Chopra has said that "Everything in life is orchestrated by an intention." In my opinion, it is really powerful to set an intention while you are preparing each recipe, putting it in the oven, bowl, etc. These are very simple, short thoughts that you state in your mind or out loud that have to do with a specific outcome you're hoping for. For instance, while rubbing chopped broccoli with oil, set an intention in your mind that this broccoli is going to taste amazing, and I mean *amazing*. Just like when you set an intention before going into a big presentation, exam, date, or race, your outcome might just improve, so do it. Speak it in your mind or out loud: "You're going to taste *amazing*." Another one is "You're going to FUEL my cells."

2: Love is the secret ingredient in every meal that you will never forget eating. It's actually written in invisible ink on every ingredient list that follows. Make your food with love, not in a hurry, with the best ingredients you can, and for people you care the most about, starting with yourself.

Are You Ready?

Let these recipes guide you, but use your instincts and your imagination too. Modify them. Enhance them. Make them your own. Create something that explodes with flavour and speaks to your unique taste buds.

Cooking is a great adventure!

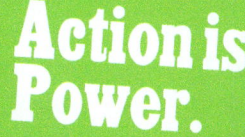

Action is Power.

FUELLED HOW-TO

Real Food Recipe Guide

Smoothies

Salads

Eat Your [Hot] Vegetables

Roasted Vegetables Rock!

Soups

Grains

Fish

Sauces, Dressings and Spreads

[Real Food] Sweets and Snacks

Cooling Drinks and Herbal Teas

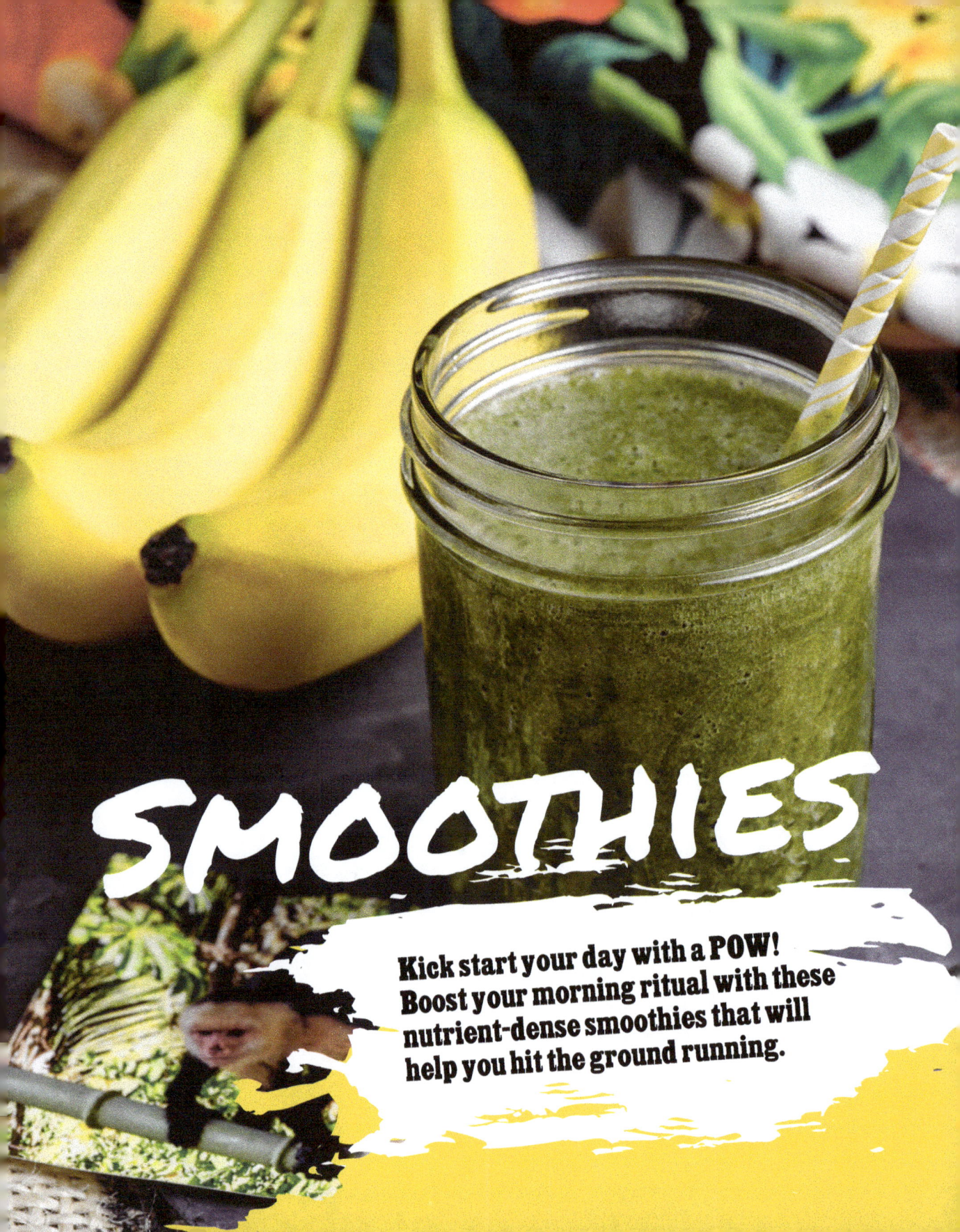

SMOOTHIES

Kick start your day with a **POW**! Boost your morning ritual with these nutrient-dense smoothies that will help you hit the ground running.

THE IRON MONKEY

Spinach & Bananas!

This is a great way to get your fresh, raw, spinach in first thing in the morning! It also makes a great smoothie bowl base. Just put it in a bowl and top with seeds, nuts or fruit.

Serves 2

INGREDIENTS:

- 3 fresh or frozen bananas, or a mixture of both fresh and frozen is what I prefer
- 1 cup spinach
- ½ green apple (a sour one like granny smith)
- ¾ cup pineapple juice
- 1 cup water (or until you get your desired thickness)
- 1 tsp moringa powder or fresh/frozen leaves if you have them (optional)

DIRECTIONS:

Blend all of these awesome ingredients in a blender until they're smooth and creamy, thick and green. Serve immediately. Enjoy!

OPTIONAL:

- Parsley – it's a superfood!
- 3 Tbsp nut butter (like almond or soynut or cashew) could be added for added flavour and plant protein.
- Substitute moringa with wheatgrass powder, spirulina, or chlorella.
- Sprinkle with 2 Tbsp ground flaxseeds or hempseeds.

The Nutty Butter Cup

Kids' Favourite!

This sweet treat boasts protein, potassium, calcium and a terrific taste! This is the only item in the entire book with caffeine—from the cacao powder.

Serves 2

Ingredients:

- 3 fresh or frozen bananas, or a mixture of both fresh and frozen is what I prefer
- 1½ - 2 cups non-dairy milk (flaxseed, almond, soy, coconut, cashew milk, etc. all work)
- 3 Tbsp soynut butter
- 2 Tbsp cacao powder
- ½ tsp raw vanilla bean powder (Optional. This can be ordered on Amazon. Use natural vanilla extract if you don't have the raw, ground bean.)
- 1 tsp maple syrup or raw honey, if desired

Directions:

Blend all of these awesome ingredients in a blender until they're smooth and creamy, thick and dark brown. Add more non-dairy milk if it's too thick. Serve immediately. Enjoy!

Optional:

- You can use a different nut or seed butter like almond butter, cashew butter, pumpkin seed butter, sunflower seed butter or even peanut butter if you want to. I generally avoid peanut butter though.

TIP: When freezing bananas, the best way to do it is to take a bunch of ripe bananas, peel them and break each one in half. Then put them in a large resealable plastic freezer bag and into the freezer. Lie them flat so that when they're frozen, they are easy to separate. I've seen so many people put an entire bunch of bananas in the freezer and then struggle to peel them afterwards! It's pretty much impossible, so peel them and break them in half before freezing.

KALE AND MANGO KOWABUNGA!

Kids' Favourite!
*when made without kale and parsley

This is one of my favourite ways to use raw kale. Makes a great smoothie bowl base. Just put it in a bowl and top with seeds, nuts or fruit.

Serves 1-2

INGREDIENTS:

- ½ cup fresh or frozen mango
- 1 cup kale
- ¾ cup pineapple juice
- 1 cup water (or until you get your desired thickness)
- 1 tsp moringa powder or fresh/frozen leaves if you have them or substitute moringa with wheatgrass powder, spirulina, or chlorella (optional).
- 3 Tbsp fresh parsley
- 2 Tbsp fresh mint

DIRECTIONS:

Blend all of these awesome ingredients in a blender until they're smooth and creamy, thick and green. Serve immediately. Enjoy!

OPTIONAL:

- For a tropical, sweeter version that kids love, this smoothie can be made without kale or parsley if you substitute 1 cup of pineapple chunks

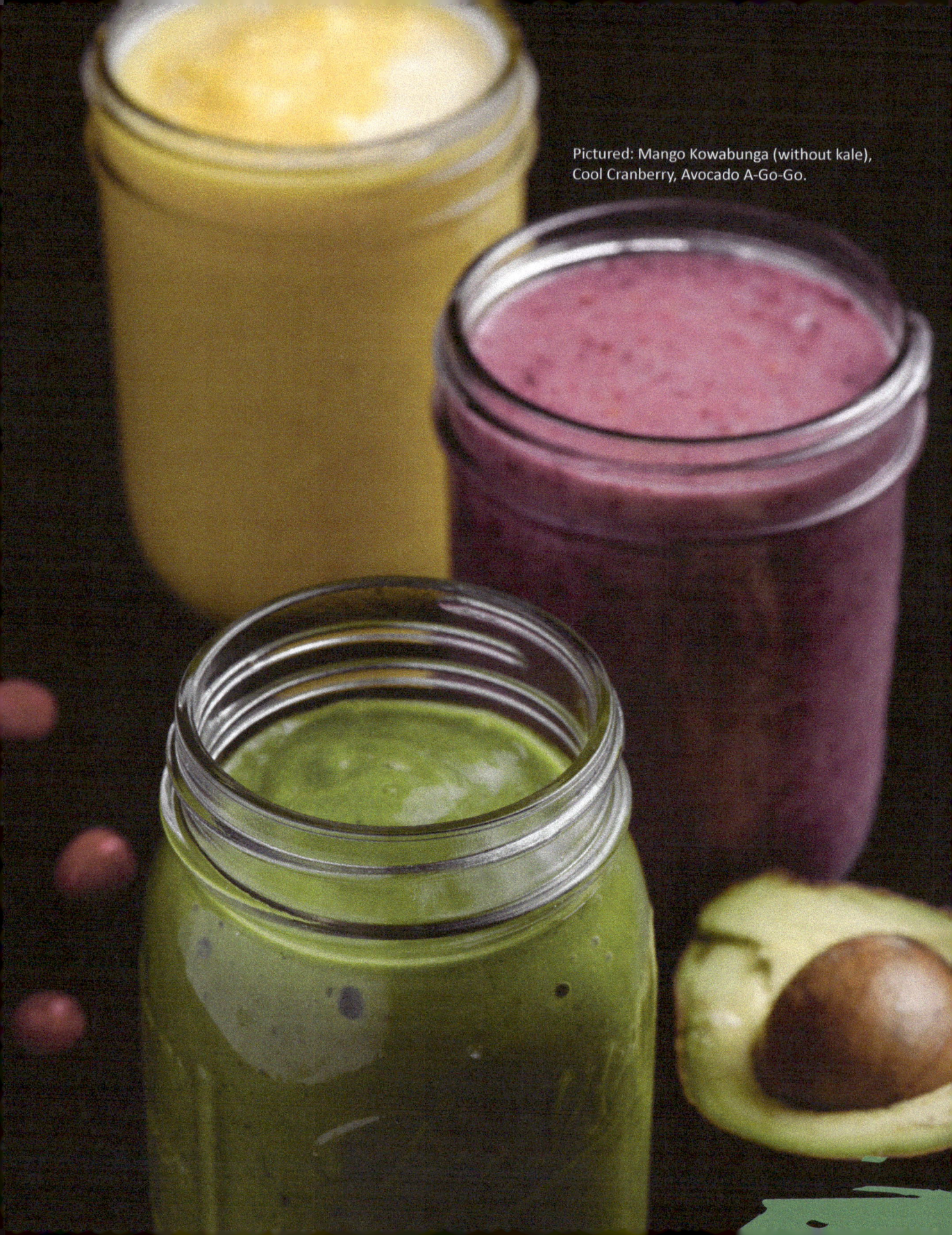

Pictured: Mango Kowabunga (without kale), Cool Cranberry, Avocado A-Go-Go.

AVOCADO A-GO-GO

Avocado is a source of healthy fat and it will make your smoothie velvety.

Serves 2

INGREDIENTS:

- ½ avocado
- 2 fresh bananas and ½ of a frozen banana
- 1 cup spinach
- ¾ cup pineapple juice or coconut water
- 1 tsp moringa powder or fresh/frozen leaves if you have them
- 1 cup water (approx.)

OPTIONAL:

- ½ green apple
- 3 Tbsp nut butter (like almond or soynut or cashew) could be added for added flavour and plant protein.
- Substitute moringa with wheatgrass powder, spirulina, or chlorella (optional).
- Sprinkle with 2 Tbsp flaxseeds or hempseeds for added fibre and omega oils.

DIRECTIONS:

Blend all of these awesome ingredients in a blender until they're smooth and creamy, thick and green. Add more water if it's too thick until you get your desired consistency. Serve immediately. Enjoy!

Maple-Laced Pumpkin Pie Perfection

Kids' Favourite!

Great in the Autumn around Halloween or Thanksgiving, or just because.

Serves 2

Ingredients:

- 1 cup canned pumpkin
- 1 frozen banana
- 1 ½ cups non-dairy milk (flaxseed, almond, soy, coconut, cashew milk, etc. all work)
- 2 Tbsp flaxseeds
- ¼ cup pure organic maple syrup
- 1 tsp pumpkin pie spice or cinnamon

Directions:

Blend all of these awesome ingredients in a blender until they are smooth and creamy, thick and dark orange. Add water if it's too thick until you get your desired consistency. Serve immediately. Enjoy!

Pear & Ginger Zinger

Serves 2

Ingredients:

- 2 cups spinach
- 1 ripe pear, seeded and chopped
- 1 cup pineapple juice
- ¾ cup water (or until you get your desired thickness)
- 1 Tbsp fresh lemon juice
- 1½ – 2 inch piece of ginger (peeled), fresh or frozen
- 1 Tbsp ground flaxseed or hempseed

Directions:

Blend all of these awesome ingredients in a blender until they're smooth and creamy, thick and green. Serve immediately. Enjoy!

TIP: Ginger freezes well so if you peel it, chop it, and freeze it in resealable freezer bags when you buy it fresh, it will be ready to use in convenient chunks for months. I add it to smoothies, use it for making ginger tea, and grate it (frozen ginger grates exceptionally well) for sautéed dishes).

TRANSFORM

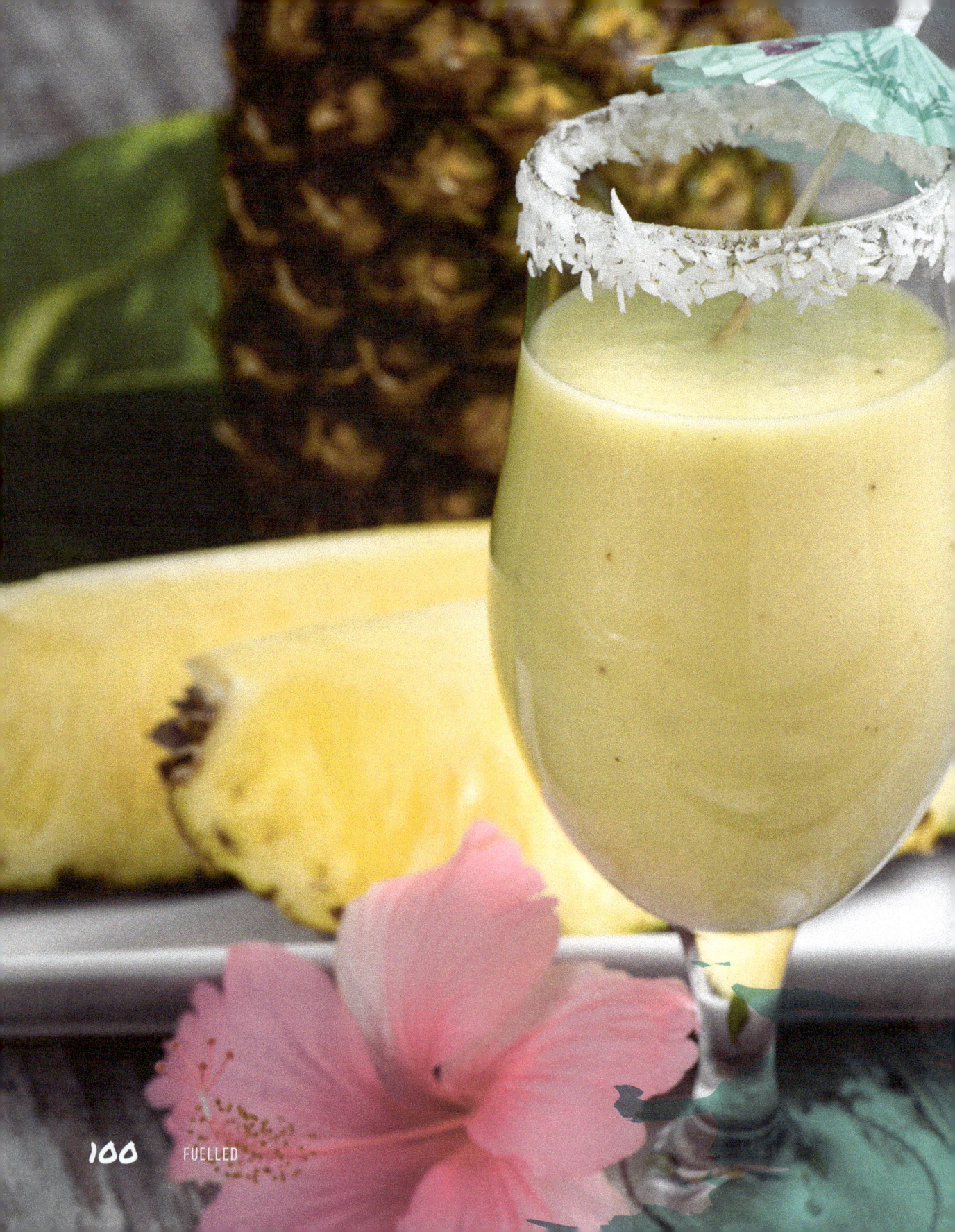

Aloha Awakening (Pineapple & Coconut)

Kids' Favourite!

This one brings the sunshine in, no matter what the weather. Make it extra special by serving it inside of half a fresh pineapple shell that has had the fruit removed from it, or in a glass rimmed with shredded coconut.

Serves 1-2

Ingredients:

- 1 frozen banana
- 1 ¼ cup fresh or frozen pineapple chunks
- ½ cup coconut milk (or any other non-dairy milk)
- ½ cup full fat coconut cream
- ½ tsp raw vanilla bean powder
- ½ cup water (or until you get your desired thickness)

Directions:

Blend all of these awesome ingredients in a blender until your smoothie is smooth and creamy, thick and yellowish-white. Serve immediately. Enjoy!

Optional:

- Add ½ cup fresh or frozen mango chunks, plus more water to thin it out.
- Add 1 fresh peach, washed and chopped, or ½ cup frozen peaches, plus more water to thin it out.
- Add 2 Tbsp of shredded dried coconut.
- Top with 2 Tbsp flaxseeds or hempseeds for added fibre and omega oils.

COOL CRANBERRY

Great smoothie for Thanksgiving on through Christmas. I love the sour/sweet combination of cranberries and bananas. Cranberries are a very good source of vitamin C, which will help boost your immune system during the busy holiday season.

Serves 2

INGREDIENTS:

- 2 bananas, fresh or frozen or mix of both
- ½ cup cranberries
- 1 cup pineapple juice
- ¾ cup water (or until you get your desired thickness)

DIRECTIONS:

Blend these simple but awesome ingredients in a blender until they're smooth and creamy, thick and pink. Serve immediately. Enjoy! Note that this does not make a beautiful green smoothie so steer away from adding in spinach or kale. It turns muddy brown when green ingredients mix in with the red berries and does not look appealing.

Tahini Vanilla Dream

Kids' Favourite!

This smoothie is so sweet and luxurious that you'd never guess it was also healthy. Tahini, the star ingredient, is rich in minerals like calcium, as well as B vitamins, is a source of protein and it aids in liver detoxification. This makes a great smoothie bowl base. Just put it in a bowl and top with seeds, nuts or fruit.

Serves 1-2

Ingredients:

- 2 fresh bananas
- 1 frozen banana
- 4 Tbsp (¼ cup) unsalted and unsweetened tahini (sesame seed butter/paste)
- ¾ tsp raw vanilla bean powder (or natural vanilla extract if you don't have the raw, ground bean)
- 1 cup unsweetened non-dairy milk (flaxseed, almond, soy, coconut, cashew milk, etc. all work)
- ¼ cup water, or more to thin it out if desired
- 1 tsp maple syrup (optional, to add more sweetness)

Directions:

Blend all of these awesome ingredients in a blender until they're smooth and creamy, thick and whitish with black speckles from all of the ground vanilla beans. Serve immediately. Enjoy!

Optional:

- Sunflower seed butter or another nut/seed butter could be used as a substitute for tahini, although tahini gives the best flavour. You can also sprinkle 2 Tbsp ground flaxseed or hempseed on top. If you prefer a sweeter taste, add a teaspoon of maple syrup, but I think it's perfect as is.

Teff Enough Smoothie

Teff is the world's smallest grain and is exceptionally high in Iron. Make a larger batch of the basic teff porridge (instructions below) in advance and refrigerate it for smoothies for the week. It hardens a bit and keeps well. You can also freeze it in portions to add to smoothies later (thawed out). This saves you from having to make it again and again as you will then have it on hand. See the Great Grains section for an amazing teff porridge recipe, another terrific breakfast idea.

Serves 2

Ingredients:

- 2 fresh bananas
- 1 frozen banana
- ¼ cup unsalted and unsweetened tahini (sesame seed butter/paste)
- ¾ tsp raw vanilla bean powder (or natural vanilla extract if you don't have the raw, ground bean)
- 1 cup of teff whole grain porridge, cooled
- 1 cup water (or until you get your desired thickness)
- 1 cup unsweetened non-dairy milk (flaxseed, almond, soy, coconut, cashew milk, etc. all work)
- 2 Tbsp organic maple syrup (optional, to achieve desired sweetness)

Directions:

For the basic teff porridge:

Pour 1 cup of whole grain teff into a pot and heat for about a minute (dry) to warm the grains up and release their flavour, stirring frequently. Pour 3 cups of water onto the teff and stir until it boils. Cover and reduce heat. Let cook for 10-15 minutes, stirring occasionally. Then turn off the burner and leave covered for 5 more minutes until it's thick but still runny, or more solid if you prefer that consistency.

For the smoothie:

Blend all of these awesome ingredients in a blender until they're smooth and creamy, thick and beige coloured with dark speckles from the ground vanilla beans and teff grains. Serve immediately. Enjoy!

The Total Daily Detox

This smoothie has ingredients that really pack some **POW!** They boost your immune system, stamina, blood flow and heart health, stimulate liver function and ease post workout muscle strain. They fight inflammation and improve eye health. They're high in vitamin C, fibre, and essential minerals like iron, potassium (essential for healthy nerve and muscle function), and manganese (which is good for your bones, liver, kidneys, and pancreas). Some of the ingredients - organic frozen tart red cherries, fresh pineapple, spinach and beets! Yes, there's a whole raw, organic, locally grown beet in there! Seize the Day. Stretch Your Wings. Give It A Whirl!

Serves 1-2

Ingredients:

- 1 raw red beet, sliced into pieces
- ¼ green apple
- ½ cup baby spinach leaves
- ½ cup pineapple chunks
- ½ cup of frozen tart red cherries,
- ½ cup pineapple juice
- 1 cup water (or until you get your desired thickness)

Directions:

Blend all ingredients in a blender and enjoy!

The Golden One

Turmeric is one of the most powerful Superfood herbs so it's a really great idea to incorporate it into your day. This is my cool and refreshing spin on the classic "Golden Milk," a potent anti-inflammatory beverage.

Serves 1-2

Ingredients:

- 1 tsp organic turmeric
- 1 tsp vanilla bean powder
- A dash of cinnamon
- A dash of cracked black pepper
- 4-5 pitted medjool dates
- 2 bananas (best if 1 is frozen and 1 fresh)
- 3 Tbsp of virgin coconut oil
- ½ cup ice (optional)
- 1 ½ cups almond milk, or half full-fat coconut milk and half almond milk
- Water, if needed to thin it out a bit

Directions:

Blend ingredients in a blender until smooth, adding a teaspoon at a time of water if needed to think it out, and enjoy!

LIGHT BANANA "MILKSHAKE"

Kids' Favourite!

This "milkshake" uses no milk but is velvety and sweet from the frozen bananas and maple syrup. It's a nice, light substitute for dairy-based sweets.

Serves 1-2

INGREDIENTS:
- 2 frozen bananas
- 1 ½ cups water
- 1 Tbsp organic maple syrup (optional)

DIRECTIONS:
Blend these three simple but awesome ingredients in a blender until they're smooth and creamy, thick and white. Serve immediately. Enjoy!

Banana "Ice Cream" Smoothie

Kids' Favourite!

This is a great substitute for ice cream.

Serves 1-2

Ingredients:

- 2 frozen bananas
- 1 ½ cups non-dairy milk (I like flaxseed milk but almond, soy, coconut, cashew milk, etc. all work)
- 2 Tbsp organic maple syrup
- ½ tsp raw vanilla bean powder

Directions:

Blend these three simple but awesome ingredients in a blender until they're smooth and creamy, thick and white. Serve immediately. Enjoy!

Optional:

- 3 Tbsp nut butter (like almond or soynut or cashew) could be added for added flavour and plant protein.
- ¼ cup of strawberries or another berry can be added.

TRANSFORM 109

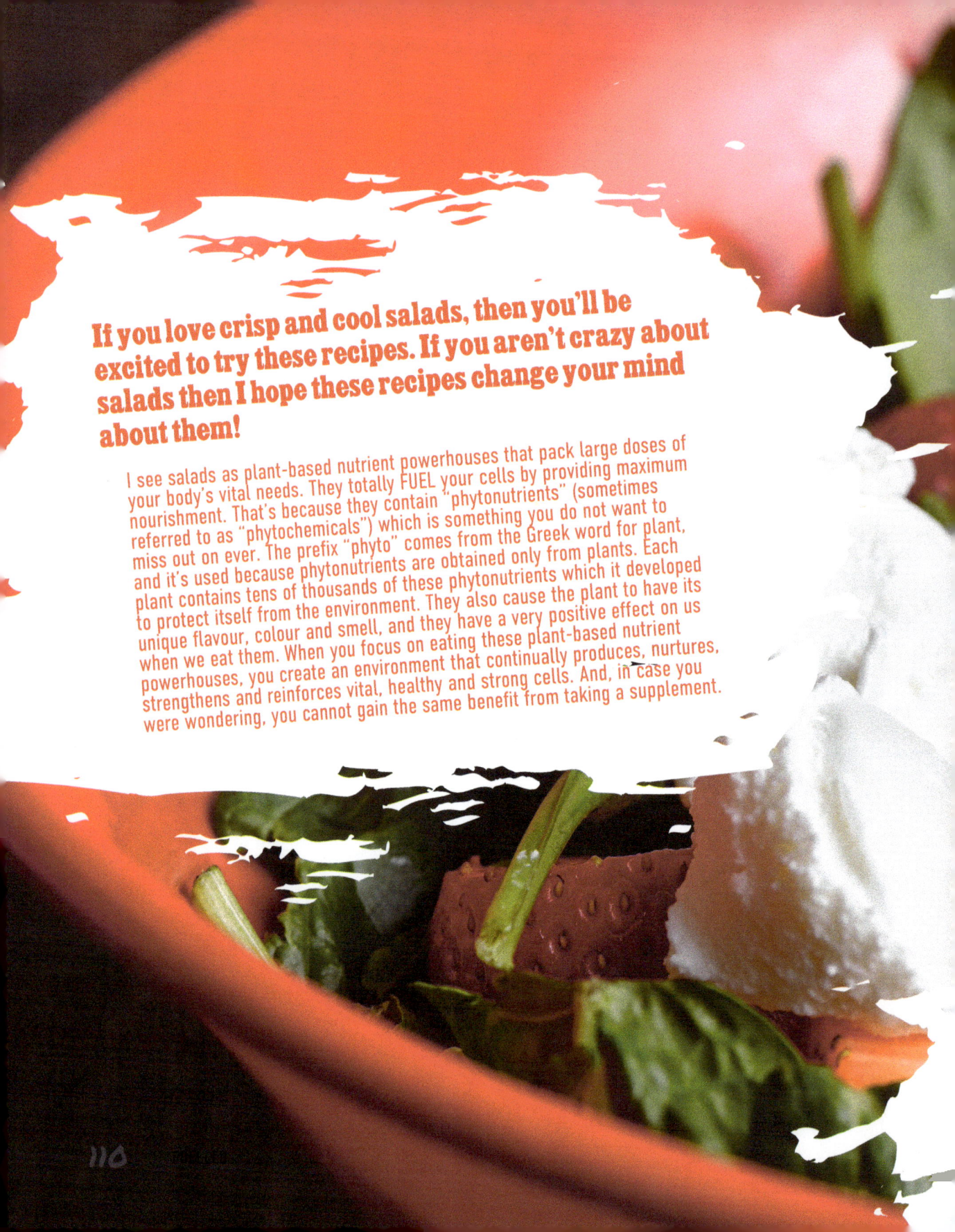

If you love crisp and cool salads, then you'll be excited to try these recipes. If you aren't crazy about salads then I hope these recipes change your mind about them!

I see salads as plant-based nutrient powerhouses that pack large doses of your body's vital needs. They totally FUEL your cells by providing maximum nourishment. That's because they contain "phytonutrients" (sometimes referred to as "phytochemicals") which is something you do not want to miss out on ever. The prefix "phyto" comes from the Greek word for plant, and it's used because phytonutrients are obtained only from plants. Each plant contains tens of thousands of these phytonutrients which it developed to protect itself from the environment. They also cause the plant to have its unique flavour, colour and smell, and they have a very positive effect on us when we eat them. When you focus on eating these plant-based nutrient powerhouses, you create an environment that continually produces, nurtures, strengthens and reinforces vital, healthy and strong cells. And, in case you were wondering, you cannot gain the same benefit from taking a supplement.

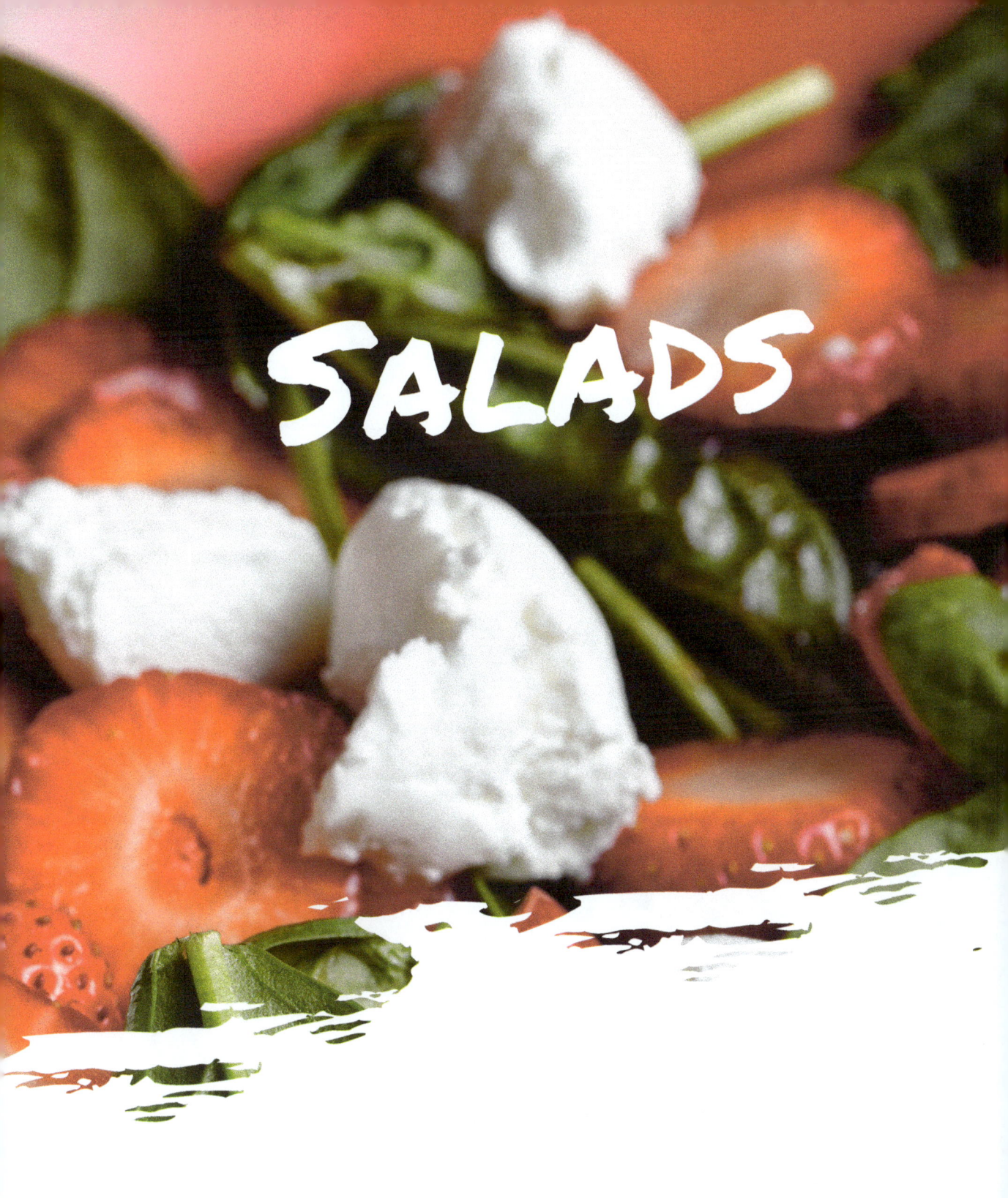

SALADS

TRANSFORM | 111

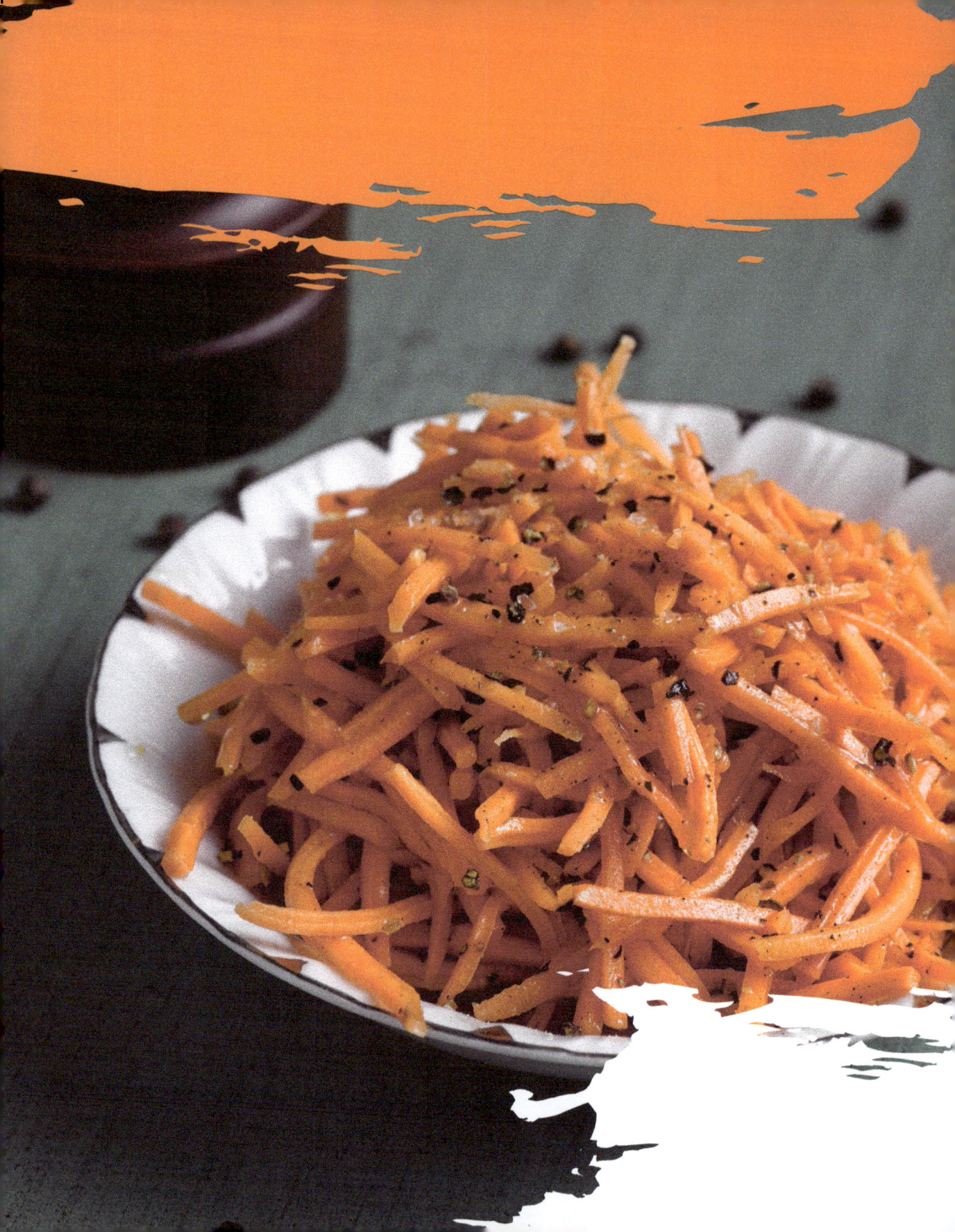

Super Simple Shredded Carrot Salad

The name says it all. It can be ready in a snap and adds a powerful kick of both beta-carotene and fibre, plus using Udo's Oil 3-6-9 Blend gives you a great dose of omega-3's and omega-6's.

Serves 2

Ingredients:

- 1 bunch (6-7) of organic carrots, peeled and grated
- 1/3 cup Udo's Oil 3-6-9 Blend or extra virgin olive oil
- ¼ tsp Celtic sea salt or Pink Himalayan salt
- A dash of cracked black pepper to taste

Directions:

Wash and grate carrots and place into a bowl. Add Udo's Oil 3-6-9 Blend or extra virgin olive oil to moisten every piece. Add a dash of sea salt and black pepper. Mix and serve. This salad stays fresh in the fridge for up to 3 days so you can make extra and pack it up for later.

Optional:

- Cumin can be added for spice.
- Sweeten it up with raisins, cinnamon, maple and grated apples.

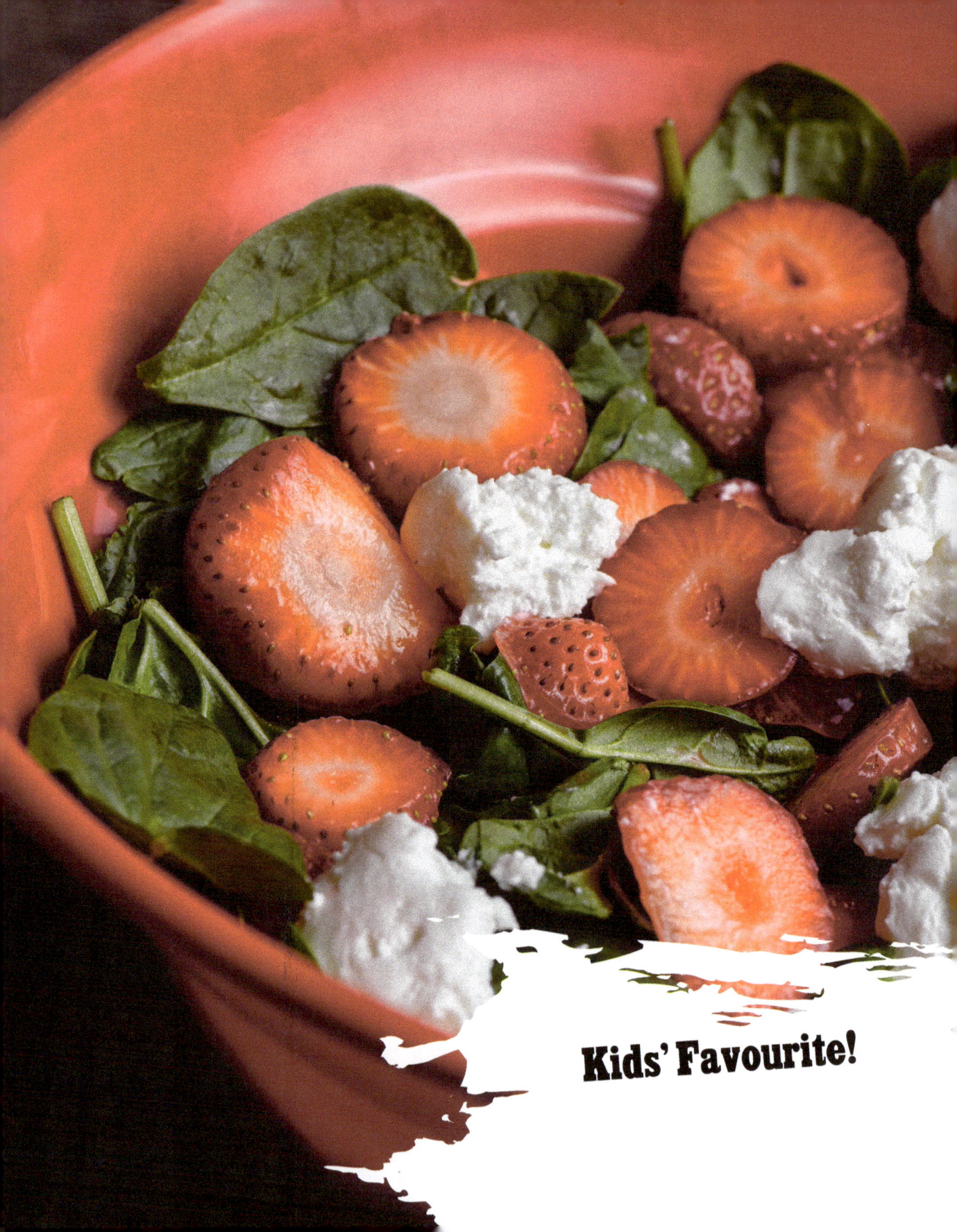

Kids' Favourite!

Spinach, Strawberry & Goat Cheese

Summer Salad

This is a crowd favourite! Bring it to a party or potluck! If it's a special holiday like the 4th of July for Americans or Bermuda Day for Bermudians, add blueberries and strawberries to the salad and make it a "Red, White and Blue Salad". Or bring the original red and white one to a Canada Day event and call it a Canada Day Salad.

Serves 4

Ingredients:

- 4 cups baby spinach
- 1 cup strawberries, sliced
- ½ cup soft goat cheese
- Aga's Fig Maple Vinaigrette (See Sauces, Dressings and Spreads, page 205)

Directions:

Toss spinach leaves with cleaned and sliced strawberries. Put small scoops/balls of goat cheese on it. Drizzle with Aga's Fig Maple Vinaigrette. Serve immediately. Enjoy!

Optional:

If you don't have strawberries, you can substitute the following:

- Raspberries
- Peaches
- Blueberries
- Sliced apples
- Sliced pears
- Dried cranberries

Plus you can add ½ cup walnuts or 4 tablespoons of hempseeds

Kale & Spinach "Caesar"

This is a great flu fighter!!

Serves 4

Ingredients:

- 1 bunch of curly kale
- 2 cups of baby spinach
- "Caesar" salad dressing (See Sauces, Dressings and Spreads, page 204)

Directions:

Wash greens and dry with paper towel. Tear kale into bite size pieces. In a big bowl, mix the kale and spinach. Pour "Caesar" salad dressing over the salad and toss before serving. This salad doesn't get soggy quickly. It can be tossed and served up to an hour afterwards because it stays crisp in the fridge.

Spinach with Caramelized Apples

Kids' Favourite!

Serves 4

Ingredients:

- 4 cups of baby spinach
- 3 Macintosh apples
- 2 onions
- ¼ cup olive oil or virgin coconut oil, for roasting apples
- ¼ cup organic maple syrup, for roasting apples
- Aga's Apple Cider Vinaigrette (See Sauces, Dressings and Spreads, page 206)

Directions:

Preheat oven to 375 degrees. Wash apples and slice into squares/chunks. Peel onions and cut them into similar sized chunks. Put apples and onions in a baking dish. Massage with cooking grade olive oil or coconut oil and organic maple syrup until glistening all over. Bake for 30 - 40 minutes. Let sit to cool a bit. The onions and apples caramelize in the oven and sweeten so beautifully. Wash greens and put in a large bowl. Place warm apples and onions over greens and drizzle Aga's Apple Cider Vinaigrette over them. Serve immediately. Enjoy!

Note: You can also store baked apples and caramelized onions in a container in the fridge for up to 2 days to enjoy the salad on another day.

Optional:

- ½ cup walnuts or 4 tablespoons of hempseeds.

TRANSFORM

Caramelized Onion Salad

Serves 4

Ingredients:

- 1 head of iceberg lettuce, washed and chopped
- 1 cup spinach
- 3 medium onions
- A dash of Celtic sea salt or Pink Himalayan salt for fried onions
- ¼ cup olive oil or grapeseed oil for frying
- ½ cup Udo's Oil 3-6-9 Blend for dressing salad
- ¼ tsp Celtic sea salt or Pink Himalayan salt for seasoning salad
- ½ tsp cracked black pepper

Directions:

Wash and dry greens, chop iceberg lettuce, and set aside in a large bowl. Peel and slice onions into rings and break apart. Coat a deep wok or frying pan with oil and sauté onions over medium heat for approximately five minutes or until translucent. Sprinkle with sea salt. Transfer warm onions onto the greens and drizzle with Udo's Oil 3-6-9 Blend. Toss all together until greens are glistening. Add black pepper and sea salt to taste. Serve immediately. By serving immediately you avoid the greens wilting from the heat of the sautéed onions. Enjoy!

Optional:

- Swap spinach for your greens of choice. I love a mixture of spinach and red leaf lettuce for texture and visual appeal.

California Cowboy Salad

Serves 4

Ingredients:

- 4 cups of greens – any of the following: baby mixed heads, mesclun greens, spinach
- 1-2 medium red onions, chopped
- 2 Tbsp smoked paprika
- 1 tsp chipotle chili spice
- 2 Tbsp of a "Cowboy rub" (steak rub) of your choice
- Dash of Celtic sea salt or Pink Himalayan salt
- ½ cup grapeseed oil for frying onions
- Goat cheese or blue brie cheese (optional)

Dressing:

- ½ cup Udo's Oil 3-6-9 Blend
- ¼ cup balsamic vinegar
- Dash of white wine vinegar (like Pinot Grigio Wine Vinegar)
- 1 Tbsp grainy mustard

Directions:

Peel and chop red onion and set aside. Coat a deep wok or frying pan in oil and sauté onions with salt, paprika, chipotle Chili spice and Cowboy Rub over medium heat for approximately five minutes or until translucent. Remove from heat and place goat or blue brie cheese on top of the warm onions so that the cheese begins to melt gently. Wash and dry greens and place in a big salad bowl. Make the Dressing: Put dressing ingredients in a mason jar and shake them up. Pour the mixture over greens and toss salad so that every piece is well coated. Top with sautéed onions and cheese and serve immediately. Enjoy!

Optional:

- Place a protein or BBQ'd/sautéed Portobello mushroom on top.

Super Spinach and Bermuda Banana

Salad with Fig Maple Vinaigrette

Ever considered having a sweet salad for breakfast? I would recommend it! This one in particular makes for a really tasty breakfast salad and you get your omega-3 in if using the Udo's Oil 3-6-9 Blend for the dressing (or hempseed oil or flaxseed oil). Give it a go!

Serves 4

Ingredients:

- 4 cups baby spinach
- 3 bananas, sliced, or 4-5 Bermuda fingerling bananas
- 1 cup walnut halves or 4 Tbsp hempseeds (optional)
- Aga's Fig Maple Vinaigrette (See Sauces, Dressings and Spreads, page 205)

Directions:

Toss spinach leaves with sliced bananas and walnuts or hempseeds. Drizzle with Aga's Fig Maple Vinaigrette and toss salad so that every piece is well coated. Serve immediately. Enjoy!

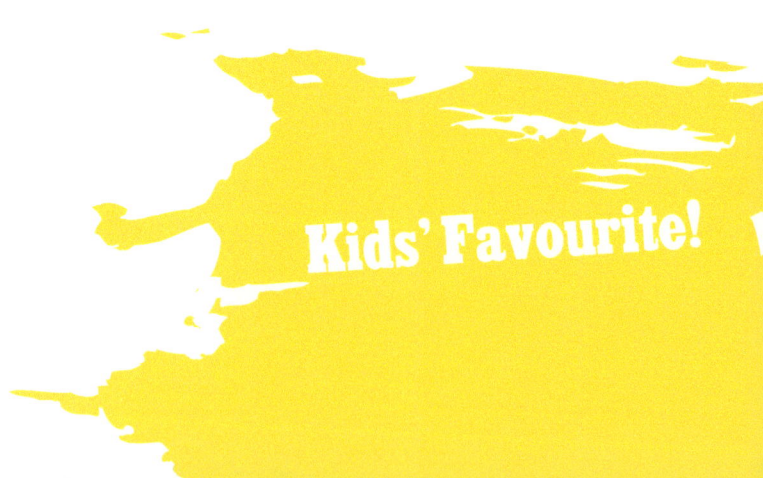

Kids' Favourite!

Roast Beet & Spinach

Salad with Goat Cheese

This is a crowd favourite! Bring it to a party or potluck!

Serves 4

Ingredients:

- 4 cups baby spinach
- 2 bunches beets any colour, stems and leaves removed
- ¼ cup olive oil for roasting beets
- A pinch of Celtic sea salt or Pink Himalayan salt
- ½ cup soft goat cheese
- Pumpkin seeds, optional as a topping

Dressing:

- ½ cup Udo's Oil 3-6-9 Blend
- ¼ cup balsamic vinegar
- 1 Tbsp of white wine vinegar (like Pinot Grigio Vinegar)
- ¼ tsp Celtic sea salt or Pink Himalayan salt
- 1 Tbsp grainy mustard

Directions:

Roast the beets: Preheat oven to 400 degrees. Wash and peel beets and slice into squares/chunks. Place on a baking dish. Massage with cooking grade olive oil until glistening all over. Sprinkle with sea salt. Bake for 45-50 minutes. Let sit to cool for 5 minutes. Prep the Salad: Place spinach leaves with small scoops/balls of goat cheese in a bowl or large dish. Make the Dressing: Put dressing ingredients in a mason jar and shake them up. When beets have cooled a bit, place them on the greens. Pour dressing over salad. Serve immediately. Enjoy!

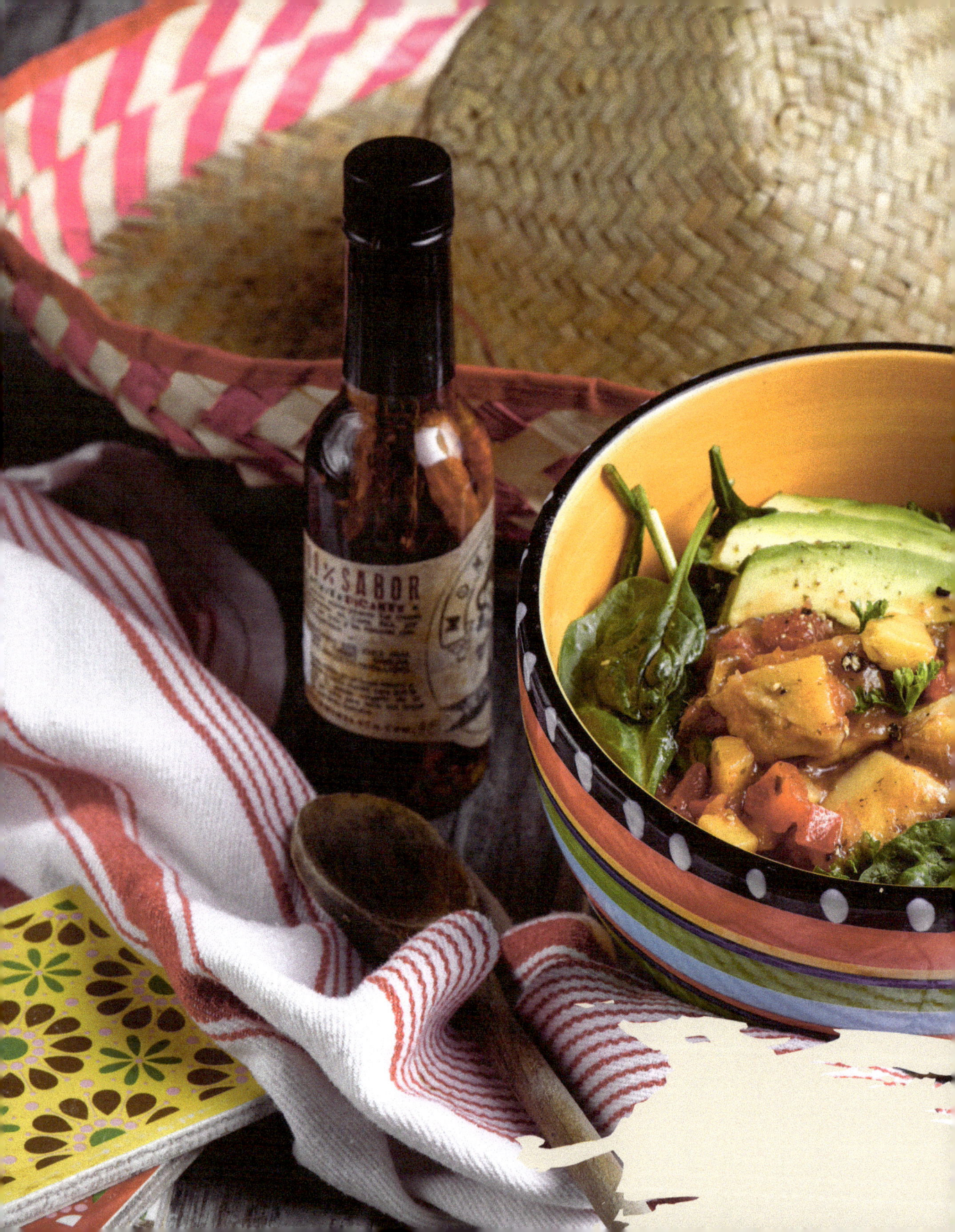

Salsa Summer Salad

Serves 4

Ingredients:

- 2 cups baby spinach
- 2 cups iceberg lettuce
- 1 cup of your favourite salsa
- 1 avocado, sliced
- 1 small red onion, chopped
- 2 Tbsp cilantro or parsley, chopped
- ½ cup Udo's Oil 3-6-9 Blend or extra virgin olive oil
- ¼ tsp Celtic sea salt or Pink Himalayan salt

Directions:

Wash greens and dry with paper towel. Chop iceberg lettuce into bite size pieces. Place greens in a big bowl and add avocado and chopped red onion. Pour salsa and oil over salad, sprinkle with sea salt and toss before serving. Serve immediately. Enjoy!

Optional:

- Ground black pepper.
- ½ jalapeño or another hot pepper, sliced.
- 1 bell pepper, sliced.

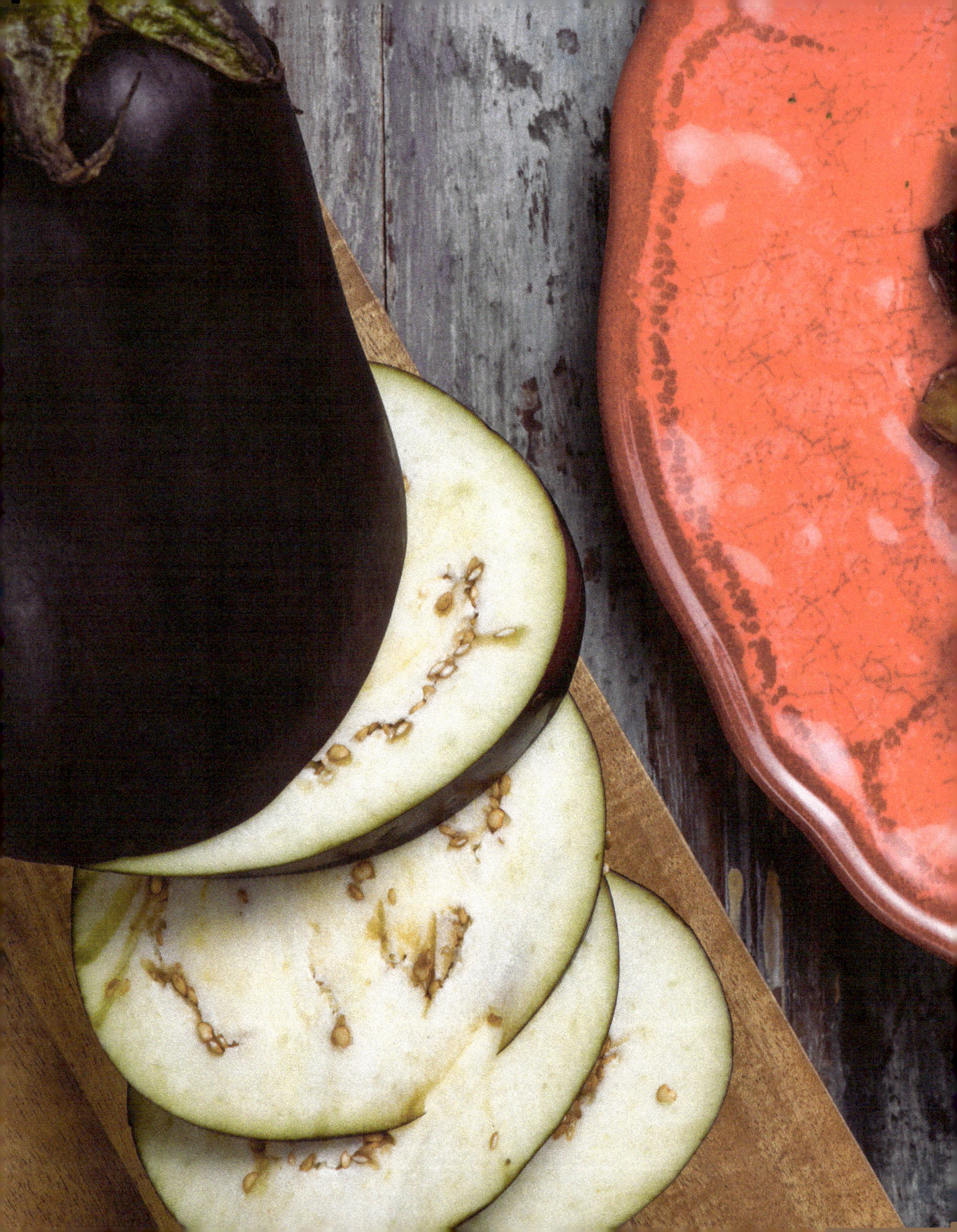

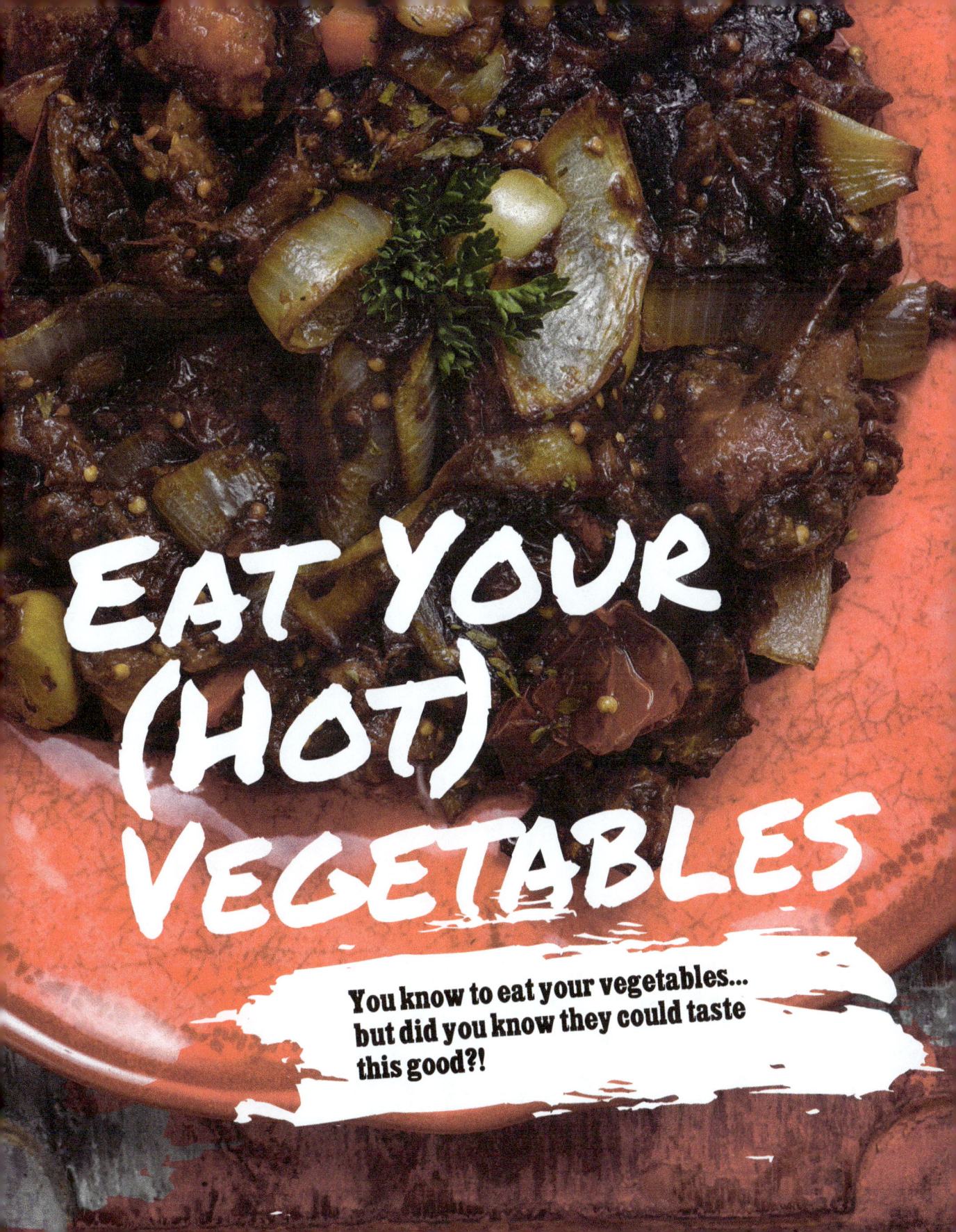

EAT YOUR (HOT) VEGETABLES

You know to eat your vegetables... but did you know they could taste this good?!

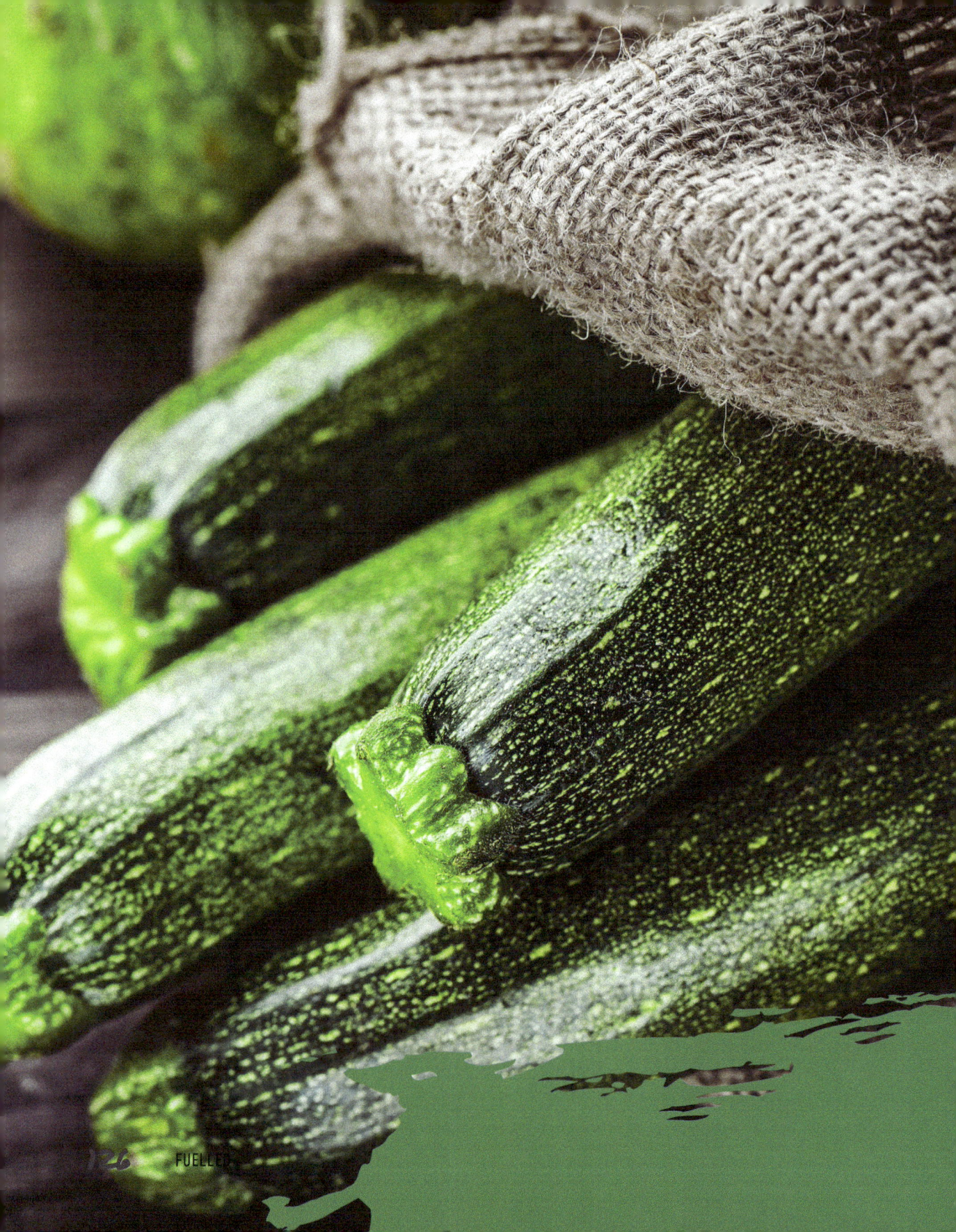

Zucchini & Leeks

Serves: 6

Ingredients:

- 6-8 medium zucchinis, diced into squares
- 4 leeks, washed thoroughly and chopped
- 3 onions, chopped
- 6-8 cloves garlic, peeled and chopped
- Exotic Roasted Vegetables Sauce (See Sauces, Dressings and Spreads, page 200)

Directions:

Preheat oven to 375 degrees. Combine chopped vegetables and Exotic Roasted Vegetables Sauce in a baking pan. Mix them around with your hands so that the dressing covers all of the vegetables. Bake for 1.5 hours, stirring at some point in the middle to make sure the dressing covers all the vegetables as equally as possible. Serve hot. These savoury veggies go very well with hot, plain quinoa or Savoury Turmeric Rice (see Great Grains chapter on how to prepare them, pages 178 and 176). Enjoy!! Store leftovers in the fridge.

CAULIFLOWER STEAKS

Kids' Favourite!

Serves 4

INGREDIENTS:

- 1 head of cauliflower
- 1/3 cup olive oil or grapeseed oil for roasting
- 2 cloves of garlic, crushed
- ½ tsp Celtic sea salt or Pink Himalayan salt
- ½ tsp paprika (optional)
- ½ tsp cracked black pepper

DIRECTIONS:

Preheat oven to 400 degrees. Wash the cauliflower and discard leaves. Slice it into 4 thick pieces, core and all. In a bowl, combine all the other ingredients except black pepper. Place the cauliflower slices flat on an oiled baking dish and coat with your oil mixture. Place into oven and bake for 15 minutes. Then take them out and carefully flip them over to the other side and bake for 20 more minutes. When ready, serve hot with sautéed onions and mushrooms on top. Sprinkle with cracked black pepper.

Easy-Peasy Greek Lemon Potatoes

Serves: 6

INGREDIENTS:

- 5 lbs Yukon gold potatoes, washed well but not peeled if the skin is clear enough
- ¾ cup fresh squeezed lemon juice (approx. 3 lemons)
- Zest of half a lemon
- ½ cup extra virgin olive oil or grapeseed oil
- 4-7 garlic cloves, minced
- 3 Tbsp dried oregano
- 2 Tbsp dried rosemary
- ½ cup of grainy or Dijon mustard
- ½ tsp Celtic sea salt or Pink Himalayan salt
- ½ to 1 tsp fresh ground black pepper (depends on how you like it)
- 16 oz chicken broth

DIRECTIONS:

Peel potatoes and cut them in half (length wise). Divide them up and put them into 2 large resealable freezer bags. Combine all other ingredients in a bowl and mix. Taste it and see if you want to add more of any of the spices. Put half of your dressing into each bag, and shake with potatoes to combine. Leave potatoes with dressing in the resealable freezer bags, place in fridge and let marinate for 2 hours or as long as overnight, whatever you have time for.

Preheat oven to 400 degrees. Put the potatoes and dressing in a large roasting pan. Roast for 1hr and 15 to 30minutes, turning occasionally. There should be sauce left over after roasting. You can put these under the broiler for 2-5 minutes to crisp them up if you prefer (I do!). Enjoy! Store leftovers in the fridge.

TRANSFORM

Not Your Mom's Sautéed Red Cabbage

Serves 4

Ingredients:

- 2 medium red cabbages, sliced and diced
- 2 medium onions, chopped
- ½ cup balsamic vinegar
- ¼ cup olive oil or grapeseed oil for sautéing, or more as needed
- 1 tsp Celtic sea salt or Pink Himalayan salt
- 2 Tbsp your favourite hot sauce
- 1 Tbsp grass fed, organic butter (optional)
- A splash of balsamic vinegar (approx. 2 Tbsp)
- A few sprinkles of cinnamon to taste
- Spices to Sauté:
- 2 tsp turmeric
- 2 tsp cumin
- 1 Tbsp rosemary
- ½ tsp cayenne
- 1 tsp cracked black pepper

Directions:

Peel and chop onion and set aside. Wash and chop red cabbage and set aside. Pour oil into a wok style pan or a regular frying pan and place over medium heat. Add sautéing spices and sauté them while stirring with a wooden spoon until the flavours and aromas are enticed out, approximately 10 seconds. Add chopped onions and salt and sauté approximately five minutes or until onions are translucent. Add the chopped red cabbage and sauté ten minutes or until soft. Add more oil so it glistens if it doesn't already. Add your favourite hot sauce, balsamic vinegar, butter and a few sprinkles of cinnamon. Remove from heat and serve hot. Tastes amazing with Forbidden/Black Rice (see Great Grains chapter on how to prepare it, page 175). Enjoy! Store leftovers in the fridge.

Candied Carrots

Kids' Favourite!

Serves 4

INGREDIENTS:

- 12 carrots, scrubbed, tops removed
- ¼ cup extra virgin olive oil
- ¼ cup organic maple Syrup
- ½ tsp Celtic sea salt or Pink Himalayan salt
- 3 Tbsp water

DIRECTIONS:

Preheat oven to 400 degrees. Scrub carrots clean under water and chop off their tops. Put into a covered Dutch oven style baking dish and drizzle with all the other ingredients, except water. Cover lid and shake the pot so all carrots get covered with liquids and salt. Open lid and add the water to the bottom of the pot. Cover and put into oven. Bake for 1.5 hours. Remove and enjoy hot. Tastes exceptional alongside the Savoury Turmeric Rice and Spicy and Sweet Exotic Rice (recipes in the Great Grains section, pages 176 and 177). Store leftovers in the fridge.

Sautéed Zucchini with Garlic & Onions

Serves 2

Ingredients:

- 2-3 zucchinis, green or yellow or both, diced
- 2 onions, chopped
- 4 cloves garlic, peeled and chopped
- ¼ cup olive oil or grapeseed oil for frying
- ½ tsp Celtic sea salt or Pink Himalayan salt
- A dash of fresh cracked black pepper to taste

Directions:

Wash and cut all veggies. Pour oil into a wok style pan or a regular frying pan and place over medium heat. Add chopped onions and garlic and pinch of salt and sauté approximately five minutes or until onions are translucent. Add the chopped zucchini and fry until soft and fragrant. Add sea salt and freshly ground black pepper to taste. Serve hot. These savoury veggies go very well with hot, plain quinoa (see Great Grains chapter on how to prepare it, page 178). Enjoy! Store leftovers in the fridge.

TIP: The vast majority of my recipes are family size because even if you're single, you do not want to be cooking a hundred times a week for yourself. Put leftovers into several containers and enjoy them a few times over the next couple of days. Freeze them so they last even longer. Cook once, eat 2 to 3 times. It's called working smarter, not harder.

Healthy Creamed Spinach

Serves 4

Ingredients:

- 4 cups chopped spinach, frozen or fresh
- 2 cups water
- 5-6 cloves garlic, mashed
- 1 Tbsp grass fed, organic butter (optional)
- 1 Tbsp rice flour (or almond flour, quinoa flour, etc)
- Celtic sea salt or Pink Himalayan salt to taste
- Freshly ground black pepper to taste

Directions:

In a large saucepan, over medium heat, combine frozen or fresh chopped spinach with water and bring to a boil. Reduce heat and add chopped garlic. Continue to cook on low heat while you mix 1 Tbsp butter in a cup with a spoon until creamy. Mix in 1 Tbsp of any flour you have as well as about 1 tsp of the liquid from the pot of boiled spinach. Mix well and then add about 1 more Tbsp of spinach water (or as needed) until it thins. Mix out the lumps and then when smooth, add it all into the saucepan with the spinach and mix together. Season with salt and pepper and serve hot. Enjoy! Tastes great with plain quinoa (see Great Grains section on how to prepare it, page 178). Store leftovers in the fridge.

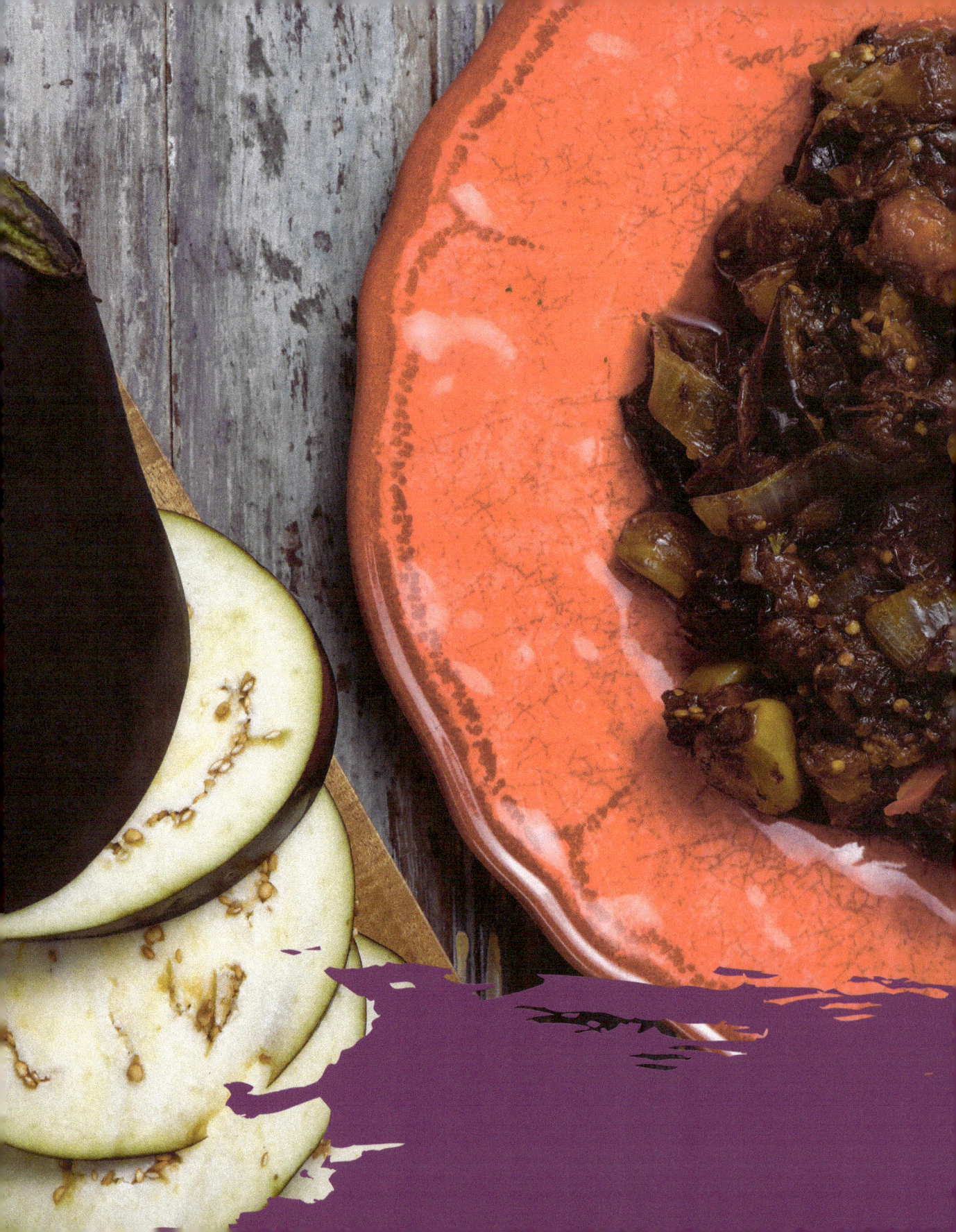

Exotic Eggplant

Serves 4

Ingredients:

- 2 large eggplants, sliced into dollars
- 2 tomatoes, sliced into dollars
- 4 onions, sliced into dollars
- 5 garlic cloves, whole
- Exotic Roasted Vegetables Sauce (See Sauces, Dressings and Spreads, page 200)

Directions:

Preheat oven to 400 degrees. Wash vegetables, leaving the skin on and place them on a cutting board and slice into circles, "dollars" (i.e., having a shape that resembles a coin) about half an inch thick. Place them into a baking pan. Mix sauce together and pour over the vegetables. There should be quite a bit of liquid. Bake approximately 1 to 1.5 hours, stirring midway. It's ready when the veggies are soft and saucy. Serve hot. Enjoy! Store leftovers in the fridge. Freezes well.

Stuffed Acorn Squash or Bell Peppers

Kids' Favourite!

Serves 4

INGREDIENTS:

For the roasted acorn squash version:
- 2 acorn squash, tops trimmed and the squash cut in half lengthwise, seeds removed
- 3 Tbsp olive oil or grapeseed oil for roasting
- Celtic sea salt or Pink Himalayan salt to taste

For the bell pepper version:
- 4-5 large bell peppers, any colour, tops trimmed and seeds removed
- 3 Tbsp olive oil or grapeseed oil for roasting
- Celtic sea salt or Pink Himalayan salt to taste

For the Quinoa stuffing:
- 1 cup quinoa (experiment with varieties: white, red or black are the most commonly found although there are 120 known varieties!)
- 2 cups water
- 1 garlic clove, sliced
- 2 cups mushrooms, sliced
- ¼ cup green onions, chopped
- 2 celery stalks, sliced
- 1 onion, sliced and diced into squares
- 2 Tbsp parsley, chopped
- 1 tsp lemon juice
- 3 Tbsp extra virgin olive oil
- A couple pinches of Celtic sea salt or Pink Himalayan salt
- Cracked black pepper to taste

For the roasted acorn squash version:

Preheat oven to 400 degrees. Rub squash with oil and season generously with salt. Place, cut side down, onto an ungreased baking pan and bake for 45 – 60 minutes, until golden brown. Take out of oven and set on stove. Prepare the Quinoa stuffing while squash is roasting and then spoon it into the squash halves so it piles up nice and high, making a bump. Reheat for 4 minutes in the oven and serve hot. Enjoy! Store leftovers in the fridge.

For the bell pepper version:

Preheat oven to 400 degrees. Wash 4-5 large bell peppers, any colour, trim the tops, remove the seeds and set aside. Prepare the quinoa stuffing and then spoon it into the cavity in the peppers so that it piles up nice and high, making a bump. Rub the peppers in oil and dash a bit of salt on them and place them upright onto an ungreased baking pan. Bake for 15-25 minutes or until peppers are tender. Remove from oven and serve hot. Enjoy! Store leftovers in the fridge.

For the Quinoa stuffing

Using a fine strainer, rinse quinoa with cool water. If you want to, you can toast the quinoa on a frying pan over medium heat for 1 minute before cooking to add a nutty taste (optional). Combine quinoa and water in a saucepan. Cover and bring to a boil. Reduce heat to a simmer and continue to cook covered for 15 minutes or until all water has been absorbed. Remove from heat and let stand for 5 minutes covered, with a paper towel in between the lid and the pot to absorb excess water. Fluff with a fork.

Pour oil into a wok style pan or a regular frying pan and place over medium heat. Add all of the other ingredients listed above for the stuffing and sauté approximately 5-7 minutes or until onions are translucent. Transfer into a large mixing bowl and add quinoa, blending thoroughly. Use this stuffing to fill your peppers or roast acorn squash.

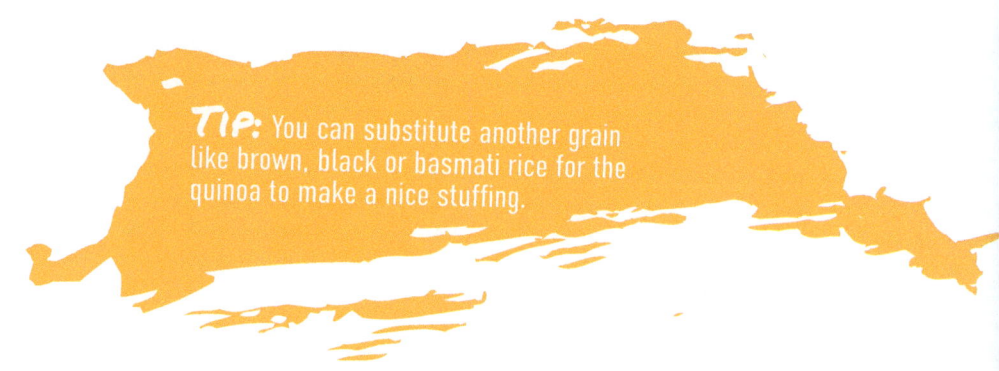

TIP: You can substitute another grain like brown, black or basmati rice for the quinoa to make a nice stuffing.

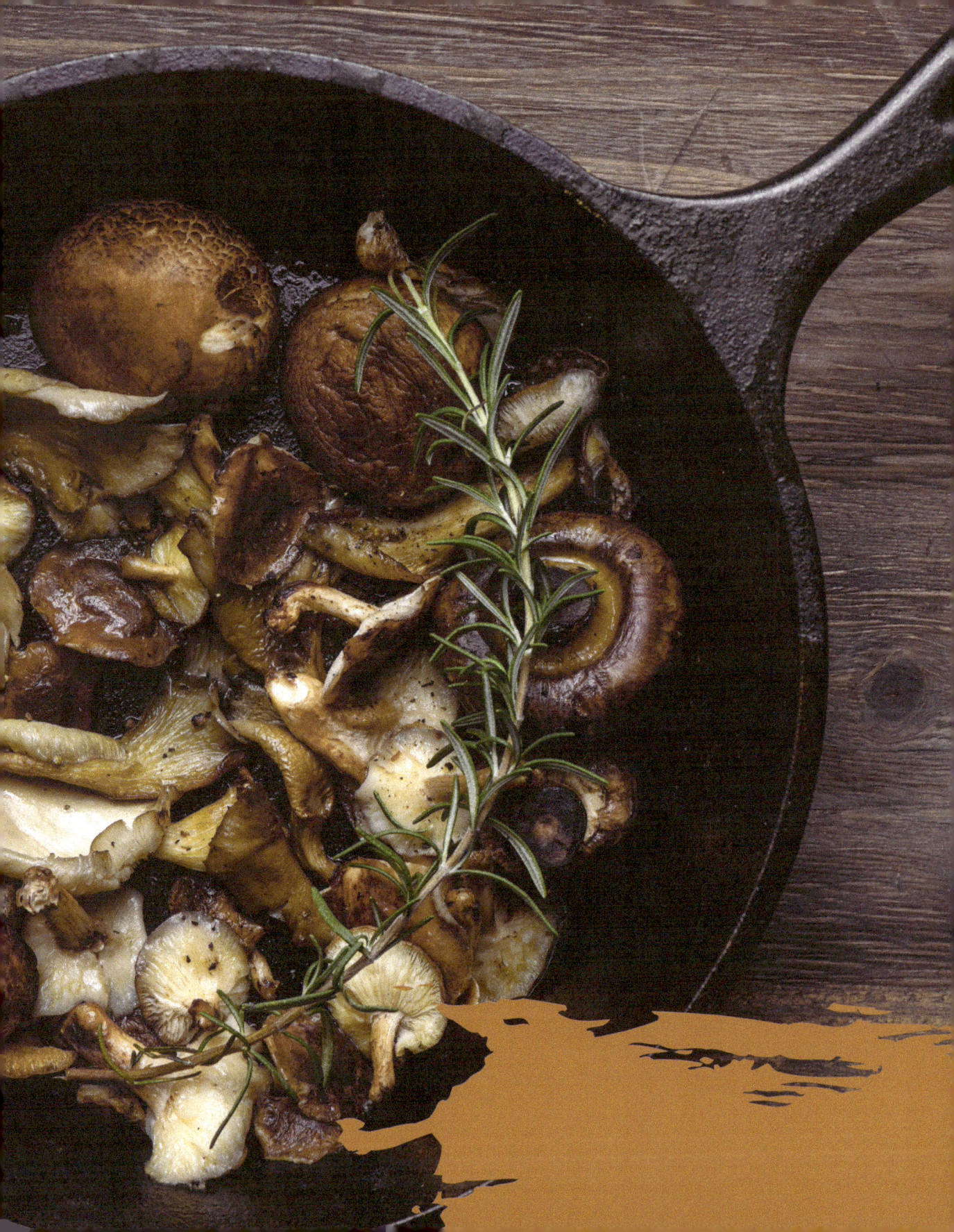

Sautéed Medley of Mushrooms

Serves 2-3

Ingredients:

- 2-3 cups of mushrooms of your choice, for example: shitake, oyster, portabella, white button
- 1 onion, chopped (optional)
- 4 cloves garlic, peeled and chopped (optional)
- ¼ cup parsley, chopped (optional)
- 3-4 Tbsp olive oil or grapeseed oil for frying
- Couple pinches of Celtic sea salt or Pink Himalayan salt
- Freshly cracked black pepper to taste

Directions:

Mushrooms tend to soak up too much water if you wash them under water so it is best to clean them with a damp paper towel or brush them off with a pastry brush. When clean, slice the mushrooms if want to (this depends on variety you use as well – the bigger, thicker ones should be sliced but the smaller thinner ones can be left whole). Chop onions and garlic and set aside. This recipe also tastes really nice without onions and garlic so if you just have mushrooms that's fine. Pour oil into a wok style pan, regular frying pan or a cast iron pan and place over medium heat. Add mushrooms, chopped onions and garlic and pinch of salt and sauté approximately 5-7 minutes or until onions are translucent, stirring occasionally so they cook evenly. Add freshly ground black pepper. Serve hot. These wonderful mushrooms go very well with hot, plain quinoa or Savoury Turmeric Rice (see Great Grains chapter on how to prepare them, pages 178 and 176), as well as the sautéed kale or garlic recipes also found in this section. Enjoy! Store leftovers in the fridge.

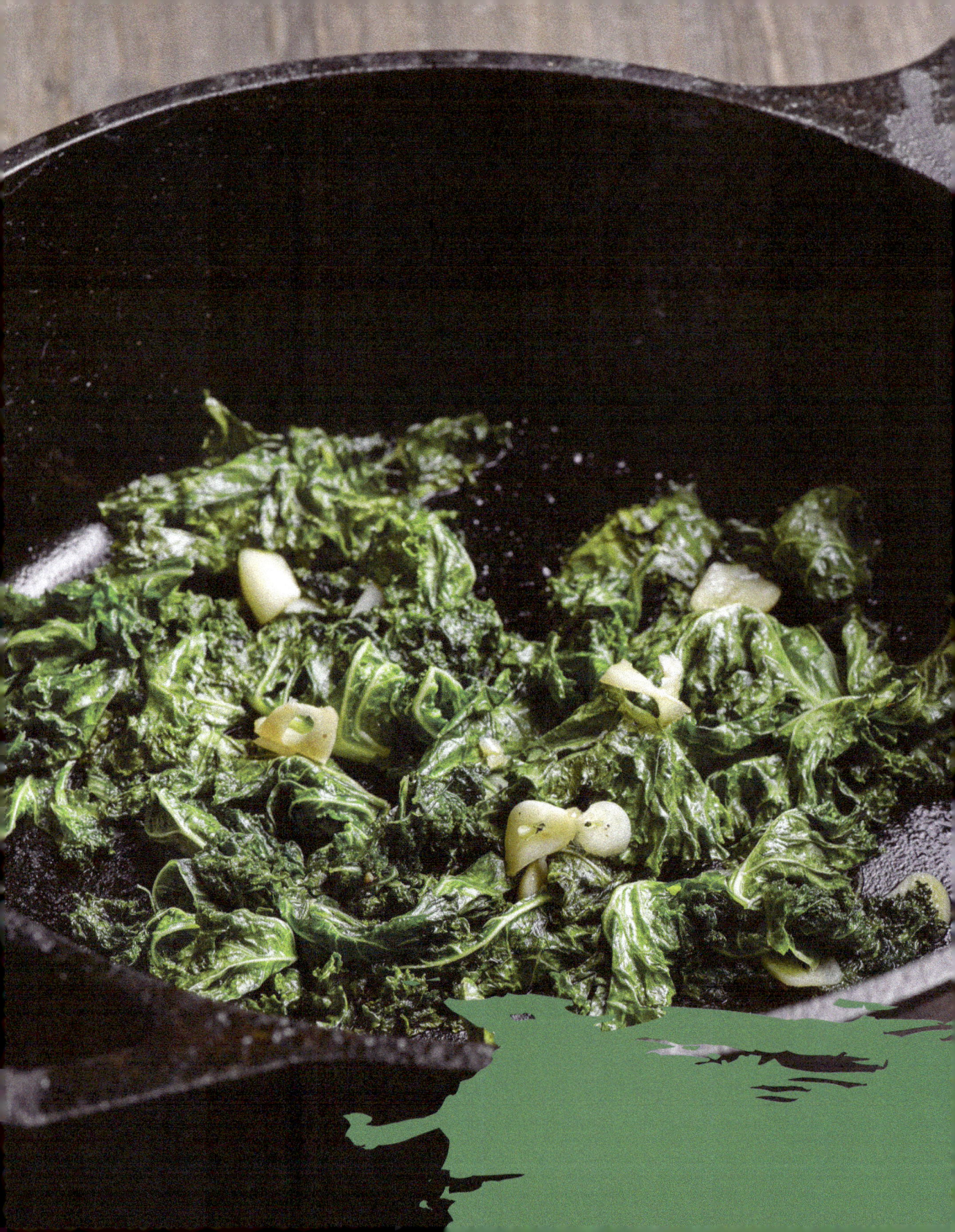

Sautéed Kale with Garlic

Serves 4

Ingredients:

- 1 bunch kale – any kind
- 4 cloves of garlic, peeled and chopped
- 3-4 Tbsp olive oil or grapeseed oil for frying
- ½ tsp Celtic sea salt or Pink Himalayan salt
- Freshly ground black pepper to taste (optional)

Directions:

Wash, dry and tear the kale leaves from the thick stems. Discard the stems. Tear the leaves into bite-size pieces and set aside. Peel the garlic and chop it up. Pour oil into a wok style pan or a large frying pan and place over medium heat. Add garlic and pinch of salt and sauté approximately 2 minutes, stirring occasionally so it cooks evenly. Add kale, pinch of salt and more oil if necessary and continue frying until kale is wilted and bright green, about 5 minutes. Remove from heat and serve. This goes very well with hot, plain quinoa, Forbidden/Black Rice or Savoury Turmeric Rice (see Great Grains chapter on how to prepare them, pages 178, 175 and 176). Enjoy! Store leftovers in the fridge.

Sautéed Chipotle Chili Kale

Serves 4

Ingredients:

- 1 bunch kale – any kind
- 1 tsp chipotle chili powder
- 3-4 Tbsp olive oil or grapeseed oil for frying
- ½ tsp Celtic sea salt or Pink Himalayan salt

Directions:

Wash, dry and tear the kale leaves from the thick stems. Discard the stems. Tear the leaves into bite-size pieces and set aside. Peel the garlic and chop it up. Pour oil into a wok style pan or a large frying pan and place over medium heat. Add garlic and pinch of salt and sauté approximately 2 minutes, stirring occasionally so it cooks evenly. Add kale, pinch of salt and more oil if necessary and continue frying until kale is wilted and bright green, about 5 minutes. Remove from heat and serve. This goes very well with hot, plain quinoa, Forbidden/Black Rice or Savoury Turmeric Rice (see Great Grains chapter on how to prepare them, pages 178, 175 and 176). Enjoy! Store leftovers in the fridge.

Smashed Roasted Sweet Potatoes with Rosemary & Sea Salt

Kids' Favourite!

Serves 4

Ingredients:

- 4 lbs of sweet potatoes (the orange ones)
- ½ cup olive oil or grapeseed oil for roasting
- 3 heaping Tbsp of dried rosemary or several fresh twigs, cut up
- 1 tsp Celtic sea salt or Pink Himalayan salt

Directions:

Preheat oven to 400 degrees. Wash and peel sweet potatoes. Place, whole, into a large Dutch oven, pour olive oil or grapeseed oil on top and sprinkle with sea salt and rosemary. Put the lid onto the Dutch oven, hold it down and shake it up so that every bit of potato is coated in oil and seasoning. Make sure potatoes glisten, if not, add more oil. Place into the oven and roast for 1.5 hours. The aroma will be incredible. Remove from oven, take the lid off and get your potato smasher and smash these up, keeping some chunks intact (you don't want it to be completely smooth). Serve hot and enjoy! Store leftovers in the fridge.

TIP: It's hard to believe but a lot of conventional spices available for sale are filled with harmful ingredients and have been sterilized by toxic chemicals and radiation. That's right, almost all conventional spices produced in the USA have been sprayed with toxic chemicals or have passed through a radiation chamber on a conveyor belt while being zapped with the highest allowable amounts of radiation for any food. This process is called irradiation and it is meant to kill bacteria, however, there are safer methods that achieve the same goal currently being used by organic producers. Food irradiation is limited but authorized in Europe, however, irradiated food or foods containing irradiated ingredients must be labelled. Try to spend a little bit extra on organic spices where you can.

If you chose not to buy organic spices, then be sure to at least read the label and don't buy any spices with the following ingredients:

- Monosodium Glutamate (MSG)
- Anti-caking agents that keep them from clumping together
- Soy and corn derivatives (these are very likely GMO)
- Artificial colours
- Artificial flavours
- Anything "hydrogenated" or "partially hydrogenated"

Also, buy smaller amounts so that your spices stay fresh and their nutritional benefits remain potent.

Sautéed Spinach with Lemon Pepper & Sea Salt

Serves 2

Ingredients:

- 4 cups baby spinach
- 3 cloves of garlic, peeled and chopped
- 1 tsp lemon pepper seasoning (or fresh lemon juice and a dash of black pepper)
- 3 Tbsp olive oil or grapeseed oil for frying
- ½ tsp Celtic sea salt or Pink Himalayan salt (double check that your lemon pepper seasoning doesn't have salt as an ingredient before you add additional salt to this recipe)

Directions:

Wash the spinach and pat dry with paper towels or spin it dry in a salad spinner. Peel the garlic and chop it up. Pour olive or grapeseed oil into a wok style pan or a large frying pan and place over medium heat. Add garlic and pinch of salt and sauté approximately 2 minutes, stirring occasionally so it cooks evenly. Add spinach, lemon pepper seasoning and more oil if necessary and continue sautéing until spinach is wilted and bright green, about 2 minutes. Remove from heat and serve immediately. This goes very well with Hot Quinoa with Ginger, Garlic and Cilantro, Forbidden/Black Rice or Savoury Turmeric Rice (see Great Grains chapter for recipes, pages 178, 175 and 176). Enjoy! Store leftovers in the fridge.

"Candied" Smashed Roasted White Sweet Potatoes

Kids' Favourite!

Serves 4

Ingredients:

- 4 lbs of sweet potatoes (the white ones)
- ½ to ¾ cup coconut oil for roasting (the mild coconut flavour turns out incredible in this recipe)
- 1 Tbsp of pure organic maple syrup (optional, depending on the taste of your original sweet potato when roasted)
- 2 Tbsp of dried rosemary or several fresh twigs, cut up
- 1 tsp Celtic sea salt or Pink Himalayan salt

Directions:

Preheat oven to 400 degrees. Wash and peel sweet potatoes. Place, whole, into a large Dutch oven, pour coconut oil on top and sprinkle with sea salt and rosemary. Put the lid onto the Dutch oven, hold it down and shake it up so that every bit of potato is coated in oil and seasoning. Make sure potatoes glisten, if not, add more oil. Place into the oven and roast for 1.5 hours. The aroma will be incredible. Remove from oven, take the lid off, and get your potato masher and smash these up, adding in maple syrup if desired, until everything is well combined but not whipped looking. Add extra sea salt to taste. Serve hot and enjoy! Store leftovers in the fridge.

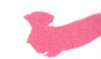

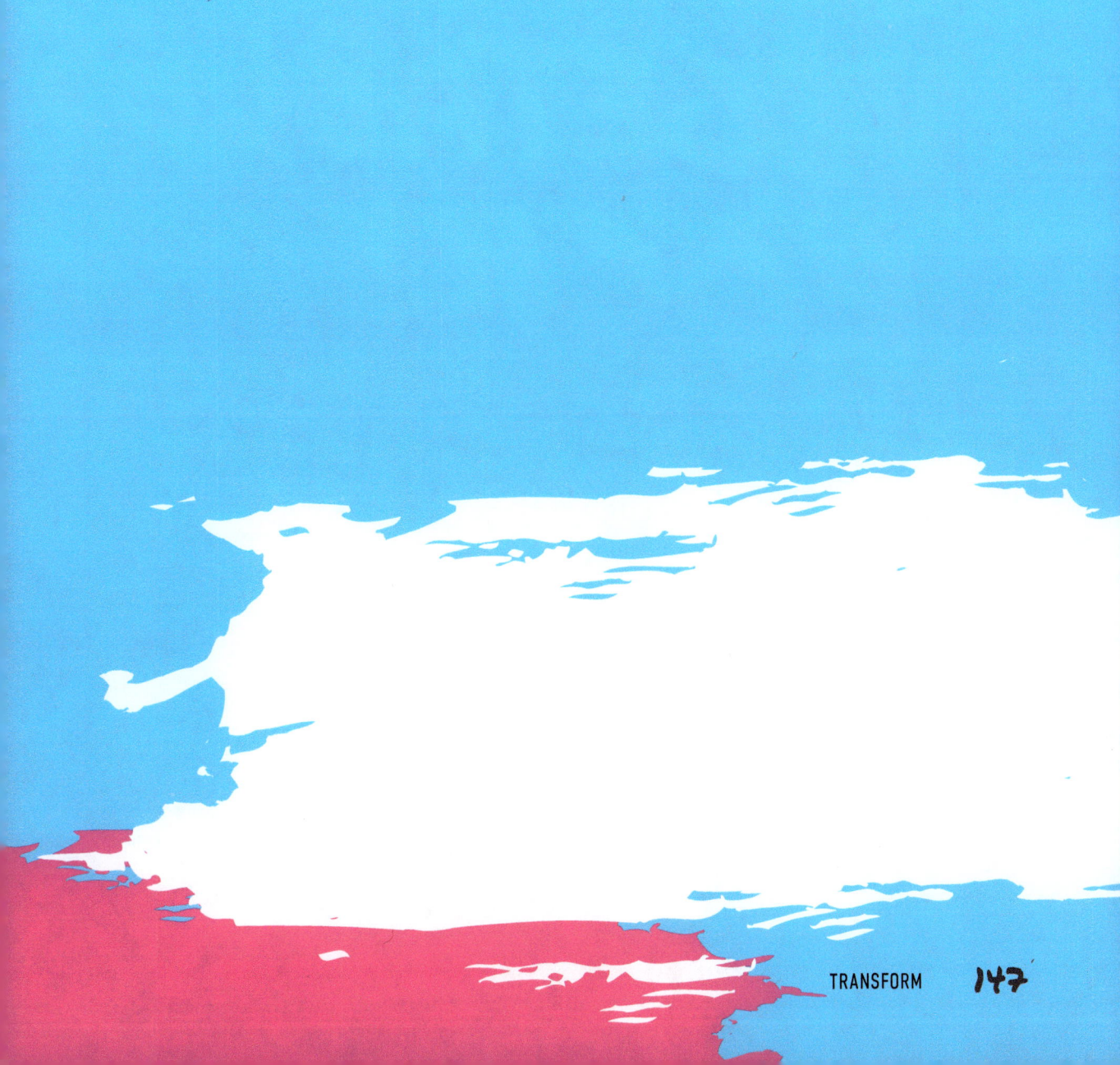

TRANSFORM 147

ROASTED VEGETABLES ROCK!

When you hear the word "Broccoli" what is the first thing that comes to your mind? Is it "Ew!" or "Do I have to…"? If so, that's probably because you've never had broccoli done right. This chapter will explain how unbelievably easy it is to create delicious roasted vegetables—like perfect roasted broccoli—that are universally pleasurable to eat and will make you change your mind forever about this green vegetable and others. In my opinion, the practice of roasting vegetables is one of the simplest things you could do in the kitchen and it'll have you eating Superfoods like they were candy. They are also a total staple in my cooking and what I consider to be one of my "foolproof foods"—real, whole foods that help support health and vitality, ensuring that I am thriving every single day. Which is what I want for you. So it's time to start making more roasted vegetables.

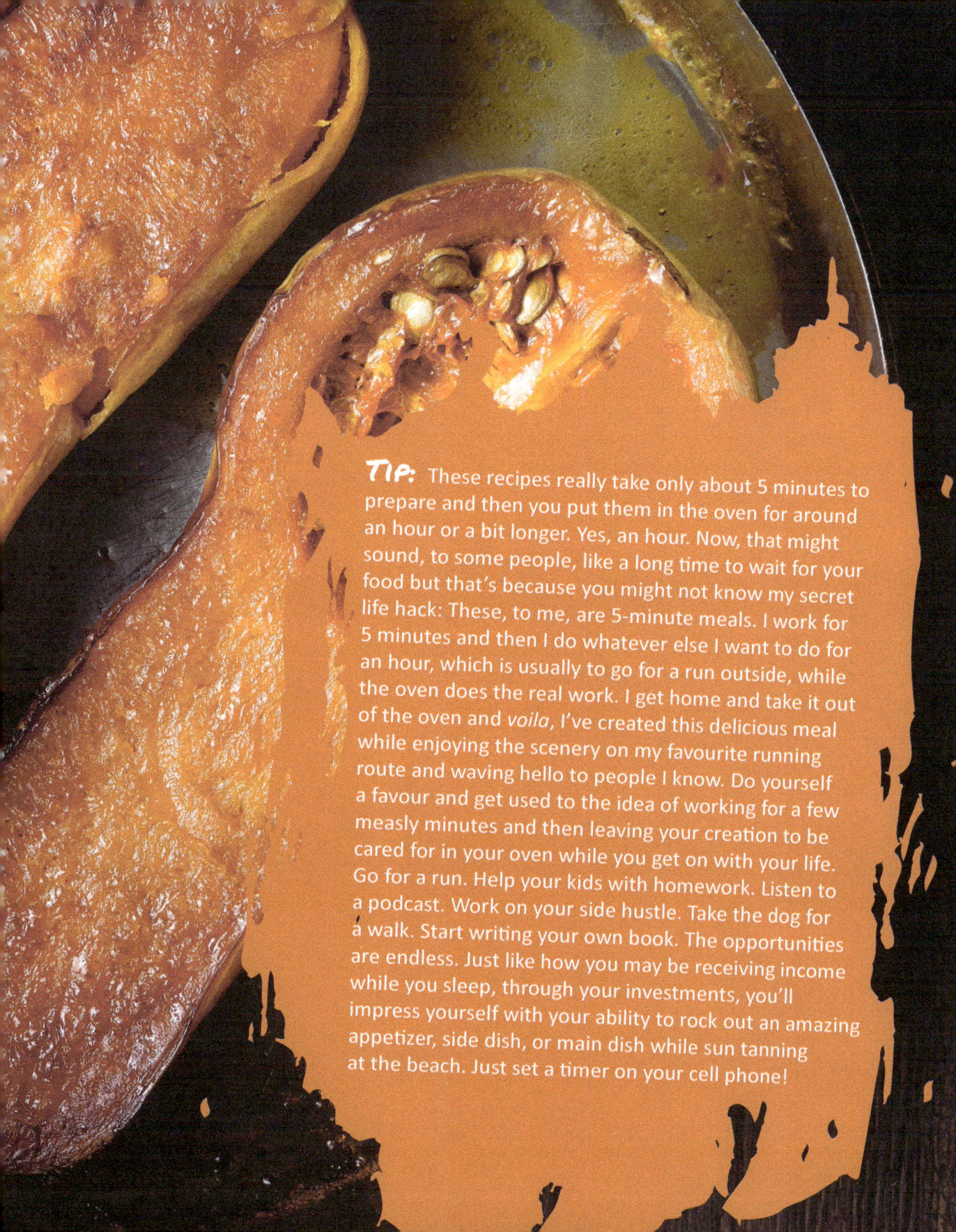

TIP: These recipes really take only about 5 minutes to prepare and then you put them in the oven for around an hour or a bit longer. Yes, an hour. Now, that might sound, to some people, like a long time to wait for your food but that's because you might not know my secret life hack: These, to me, are 5-minute meals. I work for 5 minutes and then I do whatever else I want to do for an hour, which is usually to go for a run outside, while the oven does the real work. I get home and take it out of the oven and *voila*, I've created this delicious meal while enjoying the scenery on my favourite running route and waving hello to people I know. Do yourself a favour and get used to the idea of working for a few measly minutes and then leaving your creation to be cared for in your oven while you get on with your life. Go for a run. Help your kids with homework. Listen to a podcast. Work on your side hustle. Take the dog for a walk. Start writing your own book. The opportunities are endless. Just like how you may be receiving income while you sleep, through your investments, you'll impress yourself with your ability to rock out an amazing appetizer, side dish, or main dish while sun tanning at the beach. Just set a timer on your cell phone!

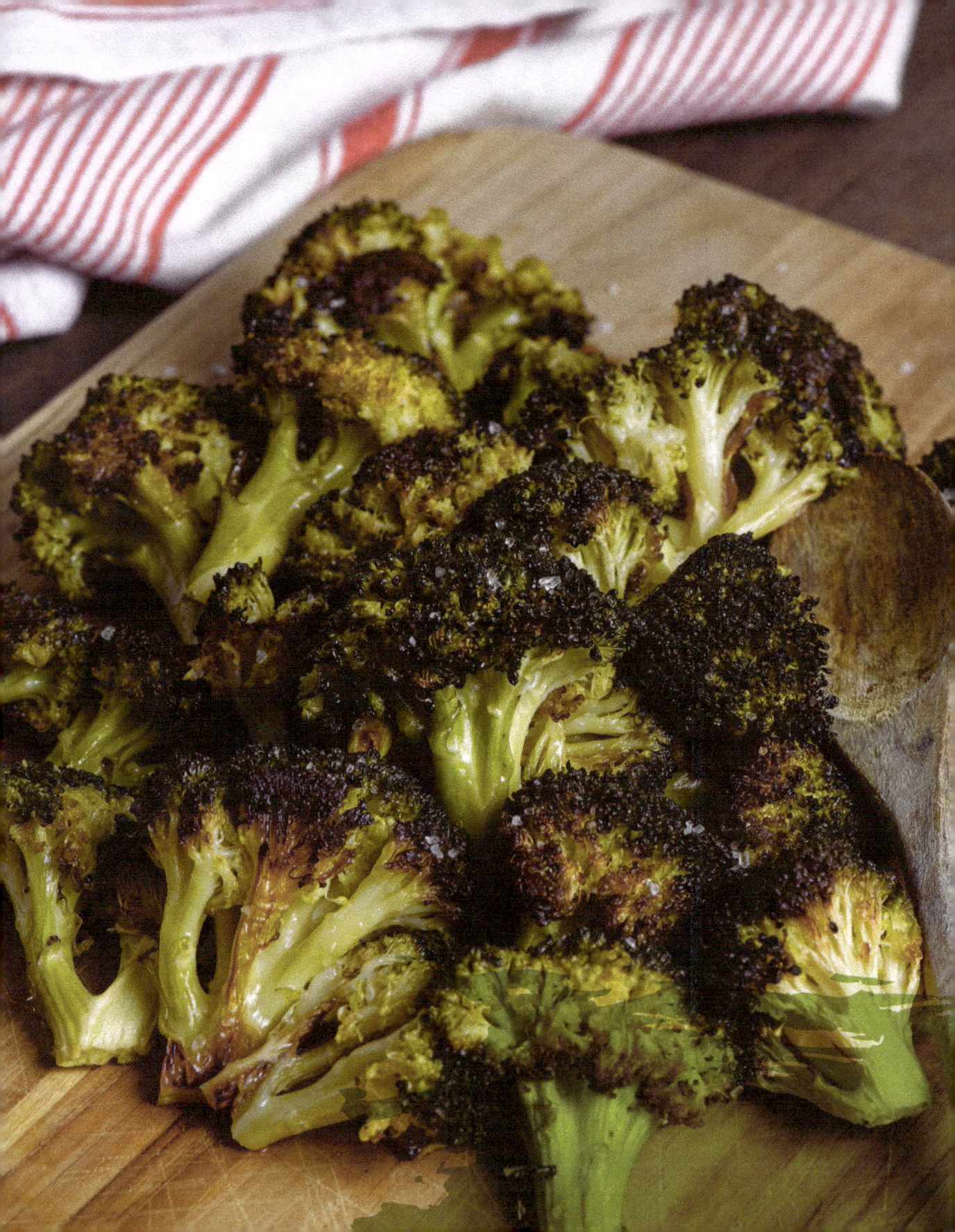

Perfect Roasted Broccoli

Kids' Favourite!

Serves 4

Ingredients:

- 3-4 heads of broccoli
- 1/3 cup of an oil that performs well in high temperatures such as avocado oil, grapeseed oil, coconut oil or an olive oil for frying
- 2 tsp Celtic sea salt or Pink Himalayan salt

Directions:

Preheat oven to 400 degrees. Wash whole broccoli, stem and all. Pat dry. Roughly chop into 1 to 2 inch chunks. Place onto a large baking pan, uncovered. Drizzle oil over the chunks. Rub the oil on with your hands so that the oil covers every part but doesn't leave a heap of oil on the bottom of your pan. Add more oil if you need to so that they are all fully coated and glistening. Do not skimp on the oil. Sprinkle sea salt on top and place into a hot oven. Roast for 45 minutes to 1 hour and remove from oven when every piece looks deep green and fried a bit at the edges. You want to see some charred bits. Do not pull them out of the oven as soon as they are tender and cooked through – they're still not finished at that point. Keep them in the oven until they reach the fullest expression of themselves. Serve hot. Unfortunately, this does not freeze well but does keep in the fridge for a couple of days. You won't have any left to freeze anyway.

Acorn Squash Fries

Kids' Favourite!

Serves 4

Ingredients:

- 2 Acorn squashes
- 1/3 cup of an oil that performs well in high temperatures such as avocado oil, coconut oil, grapeseed oil or an olive oil made for roasting.
- 1 tsp Celtic sea salt or Pink Himalayan salt

Directions:

Preheat oven to 400 degrees. Wash whole squashes. Pat dry. Cut in half so that you have 2 pieces. Then cut those in half. Then cut those into half inch pieces length wise so that they resemble fries. Place into a baking pan, uncovered, ensuring that they're not touching. Drizzle oil over the chunks. Rub the oil on with your hands so that the oil covers every part but doesn't leave a heap of oil on the bottom of your pan. Add more oil if you need to so that they are all fully coated and glistening. Do not skimp on the oil. Sprinkle sea salt on top and place into hot oven. Roast for 45 minutes to 1 hour and remove from oven when every piece looks fried a bit at the edges. You want to see some charred bits. Do not pull them out of the oven as soon as they are tender and cooked through – they're still not finished at that point. Keep them in the oven until they reach the fullest expression of themselves. Serve hot. Unfortunately, this does not freeze well but does keep in the fridge for a couple of days. You won't have any left to freeze anyway.

Irresistible Roasted Pumpkin

Kids' Favourite!

Serves 4

Ingredients:

- 1 small baking pumpkin or a 3-4 lb chunk of whatever pumpkin you have in your grocery store or farmer's market
- 1/3 cup of an oil that performs well in high temperatures such as avocado oil, grapeseed oil or an olive oil made for roasting
- 1 tsp Celtic sea salt or Pink Himalayan salt
- 1/3 cup pure organic maple syrup

Directions:

Preheat oven to 400 degrees. Wash whole pumpkin. Pat dry. Place into a Dutch oven. You can use any covered baking dish if you don't have a Dutch oven. If the pumpkin doesn't fit, cut it any which way so that it fits. Keep it simple like I do and leave the skin on. Drizzle oil and maple syrup over the pieces. Rub in the oil with your hands so that the oil covers every part but doesn't leave a heap of oil on the bottom of your pan. Add more oil if you need to so that they are all fully coated and glistening. Do not skimp on the oil. Sprinkle sea salt all over it, cover it with a lid and place into a hot oven. Roast for 1.5 hours. Don't pull out too soon. You do not want any hard pieces. It should have caramelized on the bottom parts and taste sweet, soft and comforting. Keep them in the oven until they reach the fullest expression of themselves. Serve hot. Unfortunately, this does not freeze well but does keep in the fridge for a couple of days. You won't have any left to freeze anyway. This also makes for an incredible soup base – see Soups.

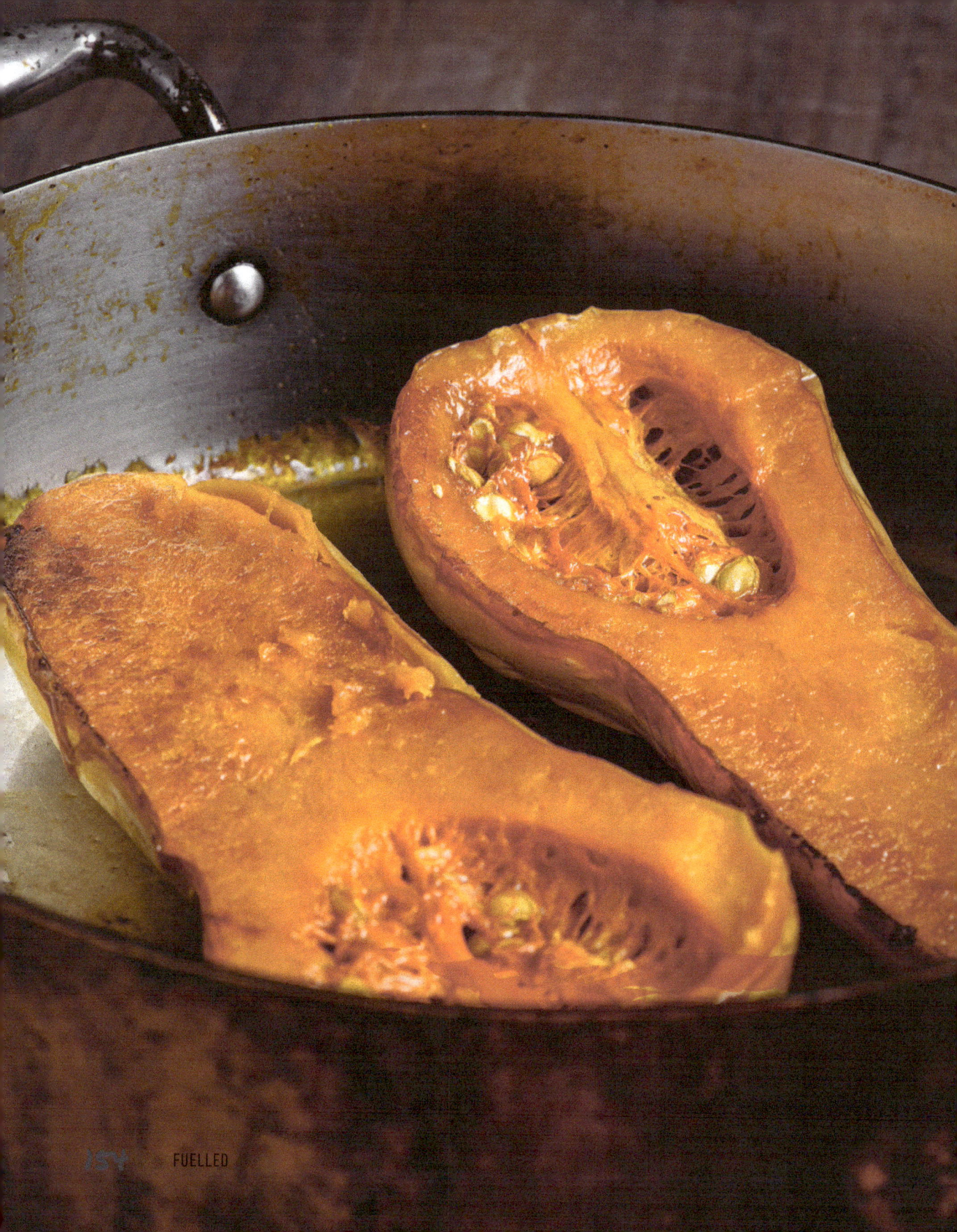

Roasted Butternut Squash

Kids' Favourite!

Serves 4

Ingredients:

- 1 butternut squash
- 1/3 cup of an oil that performs well in high temperatures such as avocado oil, grapeseed oil or an olive oil made for roasting.
- 1 tsp Celtic sea salt or Pink Himalayan salt

Directions:

Preheat oven to 400 degrees. Wash whole squash. Pat dry. Cut in half length-wise (skin on) so that you have 2 pieces. Place onto a baking pan, uncovered. Drizzle oil over the pieces. Rub the oil on with your hands so that the oil covers every part but doesn't leave a heap of oil on the bottom of your pan. Add more oil if you need to so that they are all fully coated and glistening. Do not skimp on the oil. Sprinkle sea salt all over it and place skin side up on the pan (important) and pop into hot oven. Roast for 1.5 hours and remove from oven when the top looks dark brown in parts. You want to see some charred bits. Do not pull them out of the oven as soon as they are tender and cooked through – they're still not finished at that point. Keep them in the oven until they reach the fullest expression of themselves. Serve hot. Unfortunately, this does not freeze well but does keep in the fridge for a couple of days. You won't have any left to freeze anyway. These pieces make a nice little boat for stuffing with some kind of rice or rice and meat mixture. Also makes for an incredible soup base.

Roasted Beets

Serves 4

Ingredients:

- 1 bunch beets, any colour (red, yellow or orange beets)
- 1/3 cup of an oil that performs well in high temperatures such as avocado oil, grapeseed oil or an olive oil made for roasting.
- 1 tsp Celtic sea salt or Pink Himalayan salt

Directions:

Preheat oven to 400 degrees. Cut stems and leaves off the beets and set aside if you want to use those in a different recipe later or toss if you don't want to use them (beet greens can be stir fried, added to soups and juiced). Pat dry. Cut in half length-wise (skin on) so that you have 2 pieces. Or you can keep them whole. Place onto a baking pan, uncovered. Drizzle oil over the pieces. Rub the oil on with your hands so that the oil covers every part but doesn't leave a heap of oil on the bottom of your pan. Add more oil if you need to so that they are all fully coated and glistening. Do not skimp on the oil. Sprinkle sea salt all over them and place into hot oven. Roast for 1 hour and remove from oven when the top looks brown in parts. You want to see some charred bits. Do not pull them out of the oven as soon as they are tender and cooked through – they're still not finished at that point. Keep them in the oven until they reach the fullest expression of themselves. Serve hot. Unfortunately, this does not freeze well but does keep in the fridge for a couple of days. You won't have any left to freeze anyway. I usually double this recipe at the outset. These roasted beets can be eaten just as they are or used in salads (see my Roast Beet and Spinach Salad with Goat Cheese, page 121) as well as pureed to create or enhance a dip (see Sauces, Dressings and Spreads for my Hummus recipe into which you can add roasted beets to make roasted beet hummus, page 199).

Picturesque Roasted Carrots

Serves 4

Ingredients:

- 1 bunch carrots, any colour (orange, yellow, white or purple carrots), greens left on but trimmed to 2 inches long
- ¼ cup of an oil that performs well in high temperatures such as avocado oil, grapeseed oil or an olive oil made for roasting.
- 1 tsp Celtic sea salt or Pink Himalayan salt

Directions:

Preheat oven to 400 degrees. If you bought the carrots with stems and leaves, then trim them to about 2 inches but keep them attached. Pat dry. Do not cut or peel your carrots, that's too much extra work, so just keep them whole. Place onto a baking pan, uncovered. Drizzle oil over the pieces. Rub the oil on with your hands so that the oil covers every part but doesn't leave a heap of oil on the bottom of your pan. Add more oil if you need to so that they are all fully coated and glistening. Do not skimp on the oil. Sprinkle sea salt all over them and place into hot oven. Roast for 1 hour and remove from oven when the top looks brown in parts. If your carrots are big then leave them in for longer. You want to see some charred bits. Do not pull them out of the oven as soon as they are tender and cooked through – they're still not finished at that point. Keep them in the oven until they reach the fullest expression of themselves. Serve hot. Unfortunately, this does not freeze well but does keep in the fridge for a couple of days. You won't have any left to freeze anyway. I usually double this recipe at the outset. These roasted carrots can be eaten just as they are or used in a salad.

Roasted Sweet Potato Dollars

Kids' Favourite!

Serves 4

Ingredients:

- 4 sweet potatoes, orange or white
- 1/3 cup of an oil that performs well in high temperatures such as avocado oil, coconut oil, grapeseed oil or an olive oil made for roasting.
- 1 tsp Celtic sea salt or Pink Himalayan salt
- 2 Tbsp of rosemary, fresh or dried

Directions:

Preheat oven to 400 degrees. Wash potatoes and remove any black bits with a knife. Pat dry. Leave skin on and place potato lengthwise on a cutting board and slice into circles, "dollars" (i.e., having a shape that resembles a coin) about half an inch thick. Place onto a baking pan, uncovered. Drizzle oil over the pieces. Rub the oil on with your hands so that the oil covers every "dollar" but doesn't leave a heap of oil on the bottom of your pan. Add more oil if you need to so that they are all fully coated and glistening. Do not skimp on the oil. Sprinkle sea salt and rosemary all over them and place into a hot oven. Roast for 1 hour, flipping them over at the 30 minute mark, and remove from oven when the top looks dark brown in parts. You want to see some charred bits. Do not pull them out of the oven as soon as they are tender and cooked through – they're still not finished at that point. Keep them in the oven until they reach the fullest expression of themselves. Serve hot. Unfortunately, this does not freeze well but does keep in the fridge for a couple of days. You won't have any left to freeze anyway.

Roasted Brussels Sprouts

Serves 4

Ingredients:

- 1 ½ lbs Brussels Sprouts
- ¼ cup of an oil that performs well in high temperatures such as avocado oil, grapeseed oil or an olive oil made for roasting.
- 1 Celtic sea salt or Pink Himalayan salt

Directions:

Preheat oven to 400 degrees. Wash Brussels sprouts. Pat dry. Leave whole or cut into half if you have time. Place onto a baking pan, uncovered. Drizzle oil over every piece. Rub the oil on with your hands so that the oil covers every piece of Brussels sprout. Add more oil if you need to so that they are fully coated and glistening. Don't skimp on the oil. Sprinkle sea salt all over them and place into a hot oven. Roast for 30-40 minutes and remove from oven when the tops look brown in parts. You want to see some charred bits. Do not pull them out of the oven as soon as they are tender and cooked through – they're still not finished at that point. Keep them in the oven until they reach the fullest expression of themselves. Serve hot. Unfortunately, this does not freeze well but does keep in the fridge for a couple of days. You won't have any left to freeze anyway.

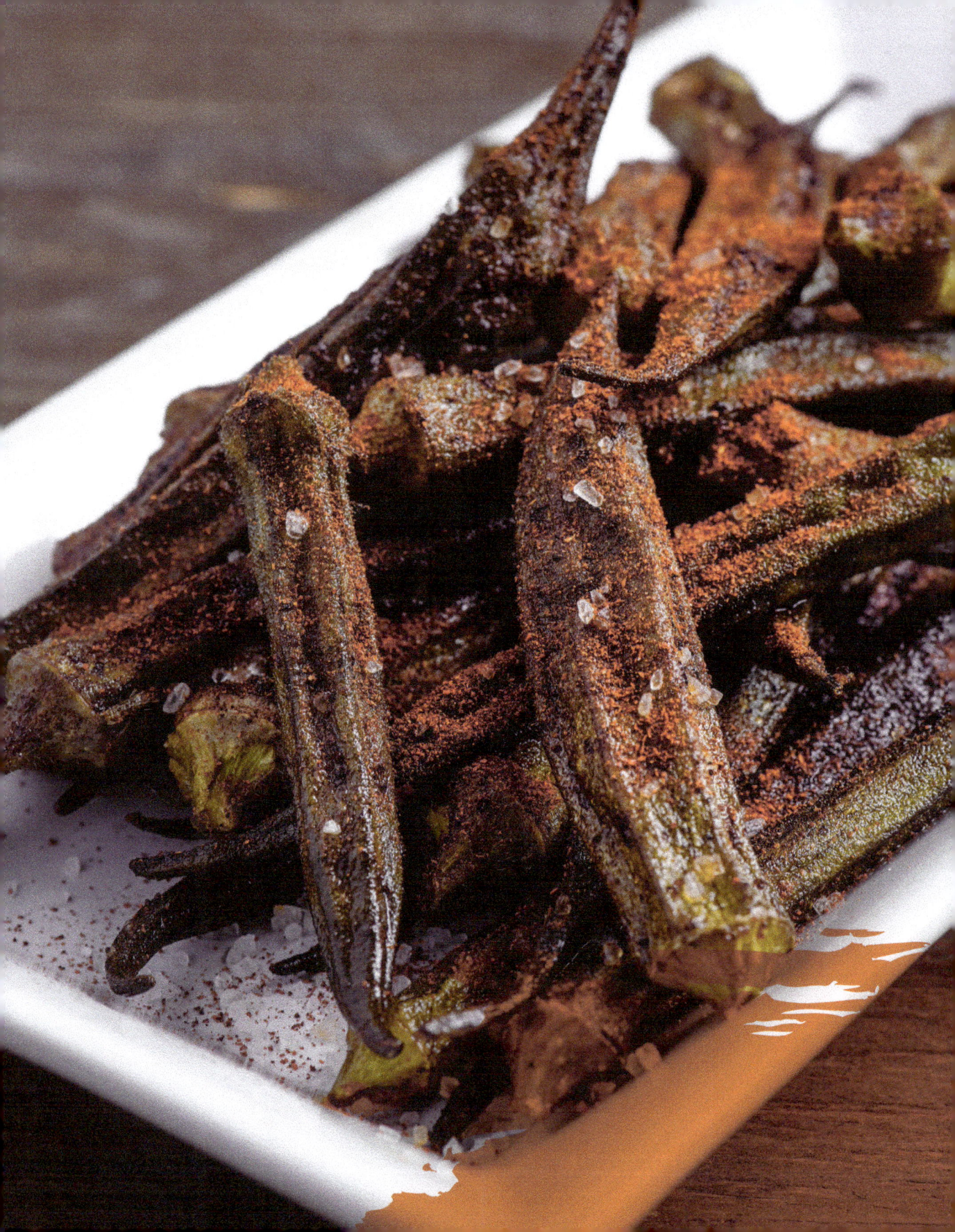

Chipotle Chili Roasted Okra

Serves 2

Ingredients:

- 1 lb of okra
- ¼ cup of an oil that performs well in high temperatures such as avocado oil, grapeseed oil or an olive oil made for roasting.
- 1 tsp Celtic sea salt or Pink Himalayan salt
- 1 ½ tsp of chipotle chili pepper spice

Directions:

Preheat oven to 400 degrees. Wash okra. Pat dry. Place onto a baking pan, uncovered. Drizzle oil over every piece. Rub the oil on with your hands so that the oil covers every bit of okra but doesn't leave a heap of oil on the bottom of your pan. Add more oil if you need to so that they are all fully coated and glistening. Do not skimp on the oil. Sprinkle sea salt and chipotle chili pepper spice all over them and place into a hot oven. Roast for 30 minutes and remove from oven when the tops look dark brown in parts. Do not pull them out of the oven as soon as they are tender and cooked through – they're still not finished at that point. Keep them in the oven until they reach the fullest expression of themselves. Serve hot. Unfortunately, this does not freeze well but does keep in the fridge for a couple of days. You won't have any left to freeze anyway.

Roasted Taco Cabbage

Serves 2

Ingredients:

- 1 large green or red cabbage or 2 medium/small sized cabbages
- ¼ cup of an oil that performs well in high temperatures such as avocado oil, grapeseed oil or an olive oil made for roasting.
- 1 package of your favourite taco seasoning, or more to taste (check ingredients to make sure it doesn't include chemicals or flour or other ingredients that aren't spices).

Directions:

Preheat oven to 400 degrees. Wash cabbage. Pat dry. Cut in half length-wise so that you have 2 pieces. Then go to town chopping it up into half inch thick slices/parts. Place onto a baking pan, uncovered. Drizzle oil over all of the pieces. Rub the oil on with your hands so that the oil covers every part but doesn't leave a heap of oil on the bottom of your pan. Add more oil if you need to so that it is all fully coated and glistening. Do not skimp on the oil. Sprinkle taco seasoning all over it and place into hot oven. Roast for 45 minutes and remove from oven when the top looks brown in parts. You want to see some charred bits. Do not pull them out of the oven as soon as they are tender and cooked through – they're still not finished at that point. Keep them in the oven until they reach the fullest expression of themselves. Serve hot. This freezes well and keeps in the fridge for a couple of days.

Medley of Roasted Vegetables

If you want to create a colourful medley of roasted vegetables, prepare some roasted carrots, Brussels sprouts, broccoli, cauliflower, acorn squash, sweet potatoes and beets (or whatever you enjoy the most) individually and cut them into small 1 inch pieces when done and combine together in a bowl or baking dish. Serve hot. Feel free to add your favourite spice to all of them when roasting them so that your medley has extra flavours. I would recommend rosemary, parsley, thyme or a bit of marjoram. Add feta or goat cheese on top if you'd like.

You Can Roast Any Vegetable

You will notice that the same procedure is used over and over again in the recipes above. Once you get the hang of roasting these vegetables, try experimenting with any vegetable you enjoy—from turnips to red peppers to cauliflower to asparagus to onions to tomatoes to garlic to Portobello mushrooms. I have no doubt that you will find all of them incredibly pleasurable to eat.

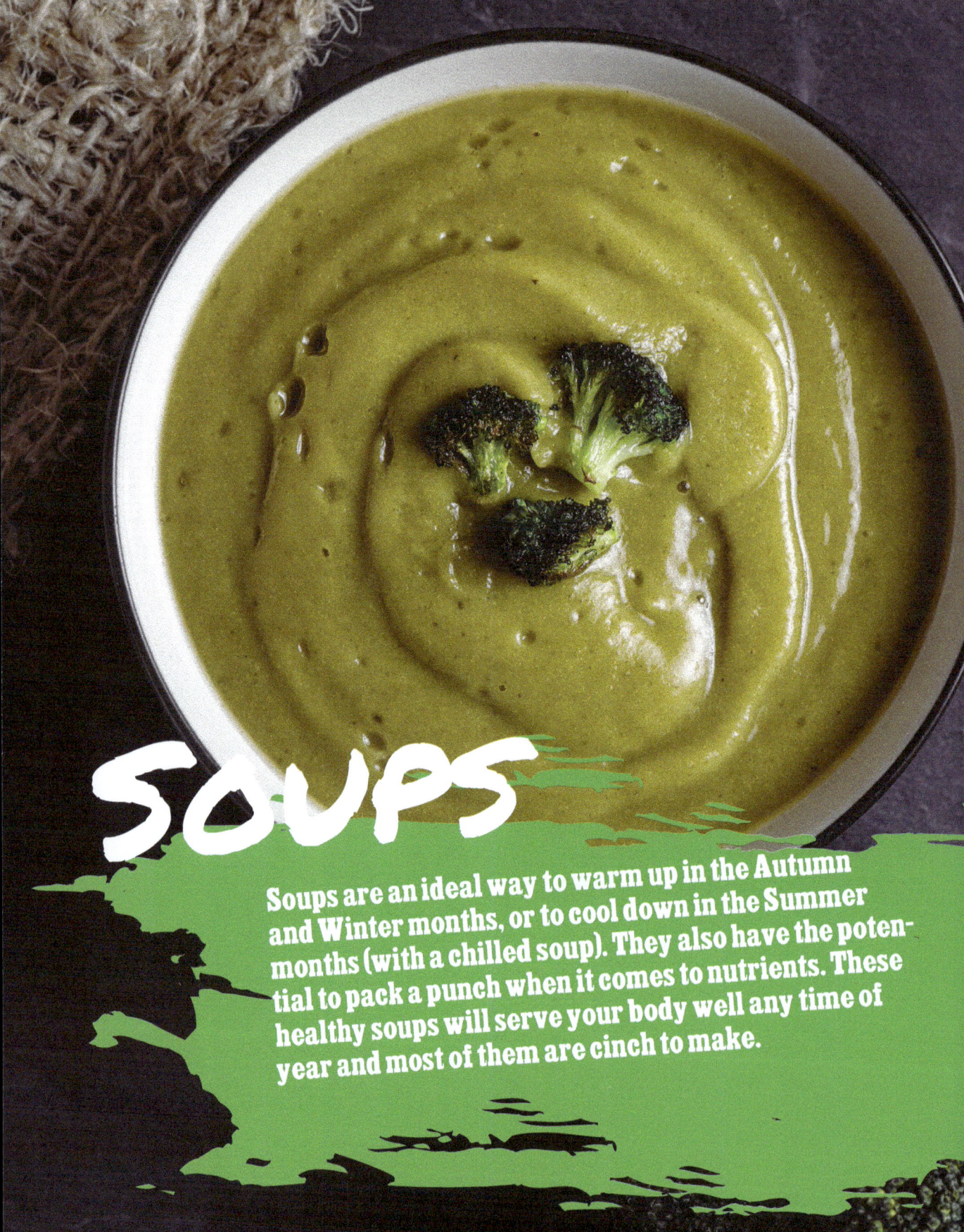

SOUPS

Soups are an ideal way to warm up in the Autumn and Winter months, or to cool down in the Summer months (with a chilled soup). They also have the potential to pack a punch when it comes to nutrients. These healthy soups will serve your body well any time of year and most of them are cinch to make.

3-Ingredient Creamy Broccoli Soup

Serves 2

Ingredients:

- 2 big heads of broccoli (I use the whole broccoli – stems, leaves and all)
- 3 Tbsp Bragg's Liquid Aminos
- Pinch of garlic powder
- Water

Directions:

Wash the broccoli and place it in a steamer basket over a large pot on high heat. Steam for approximately 30 minutes or until soft. Remove broccoli from heat and place into a blender with enough water to cover the top of the broccoli. Blend until smooth. This may take a few rounds in the blender. During one of the rounds, add Bragg's Liquid Aminos and garlic powder and blend until creamy. Pour all of the soup into a large soup pot, stir together so that the seasoning is evenly distributed, reheat and serve. Store leftovers in the fridge up to 2 days. This soup doesn't do well in the freezer.

Simplest Borscht Ever

Serves 8

Ingredients:

- 8 beets, peeled and chopped in half, and a few beet leaves
- 16-18 cups of water
- 4 carrots
- 6-8 cloves of garlic
- 2 onions, chopped
- ½ bunch of kale (optional)
- ½ bunch of parsley, chopped
- 2 tsp Celtic sea salt or Pink Himalayan salt
- 2 tsp fresh cracked black pepper
- A splash of balsamic vinegar (approx. 3 Tbsp)

Directions:

Fill a large soup pot with 16-18 cups of water. Wash, peel and chop beets, beet leaves, carrots, kale, parsley and onions. Place all vegetables into your large soup pot, ensuring all vegetables are fully submerged. Add salt and pepper. Bring to a boil on high heat, then reduce heat to medium and cook for 1 hour, with pot lid cracked open a little bit to release steam. About 45 minutes in, add splash of balsamic vinegar. Adjust seasoning to taste. Serve hot. Store leftovers in the fridge. Freezes well.

Fish Taco Soup with Garden Vegetables

Serves 6-8

INGREDIENTS:

- 2 lbs white fish, preferably a type of fish listed under "Best Choices" or "Good Alternatives" on the Monterey Bay Aquarium Seafood Watch Consumer Guide (See the Seafood section in Section 1 of this book)
- 16-18 cups of water
- 4 Tbsp olive oil or grapeseed oil
- 4 packages of your favourite Taco Seasoning (read the label carefully to ensure it doesn't include flour, corn products or hydrogenated oils).
- 3 onions, chopped
- 6 cloves of garlic, chopped
- 1 bunch parsley, chopped
- 2 cups of raw green beans
- 2 lbs of pumpkin, cut into cubes
- ½ small cabbage, chopped
- 4 carrots, cut into dollars
- 2 tsp Celtic sea salt or Pink Himalayan salt
- 1 Tbsp dried parsley
- A splash of balsamic vinegar, to taste (approx. 3 Tbsp)
- A pinch of cracked black pepper

DIRECTIONS:

Coat the bottom of a large soup pot with oil and add your favourite Taco seasoning, chopped onions and fish filets. Put on medium heat and sauté until you release the aromas, approximately 1 minute. Add more oil as needed. Add water. Add all of the rest of the vegetables and chopped parsley. Add sea salt and dried parsley. Bring to a boil and then lower heat to medium and cook for approximately 1 hour, with the lid partially open to allow steam out. Spike with balsamic vinegar and pinch of cracked black pepper to taste and serve hot. Store leftovers in the fridge.

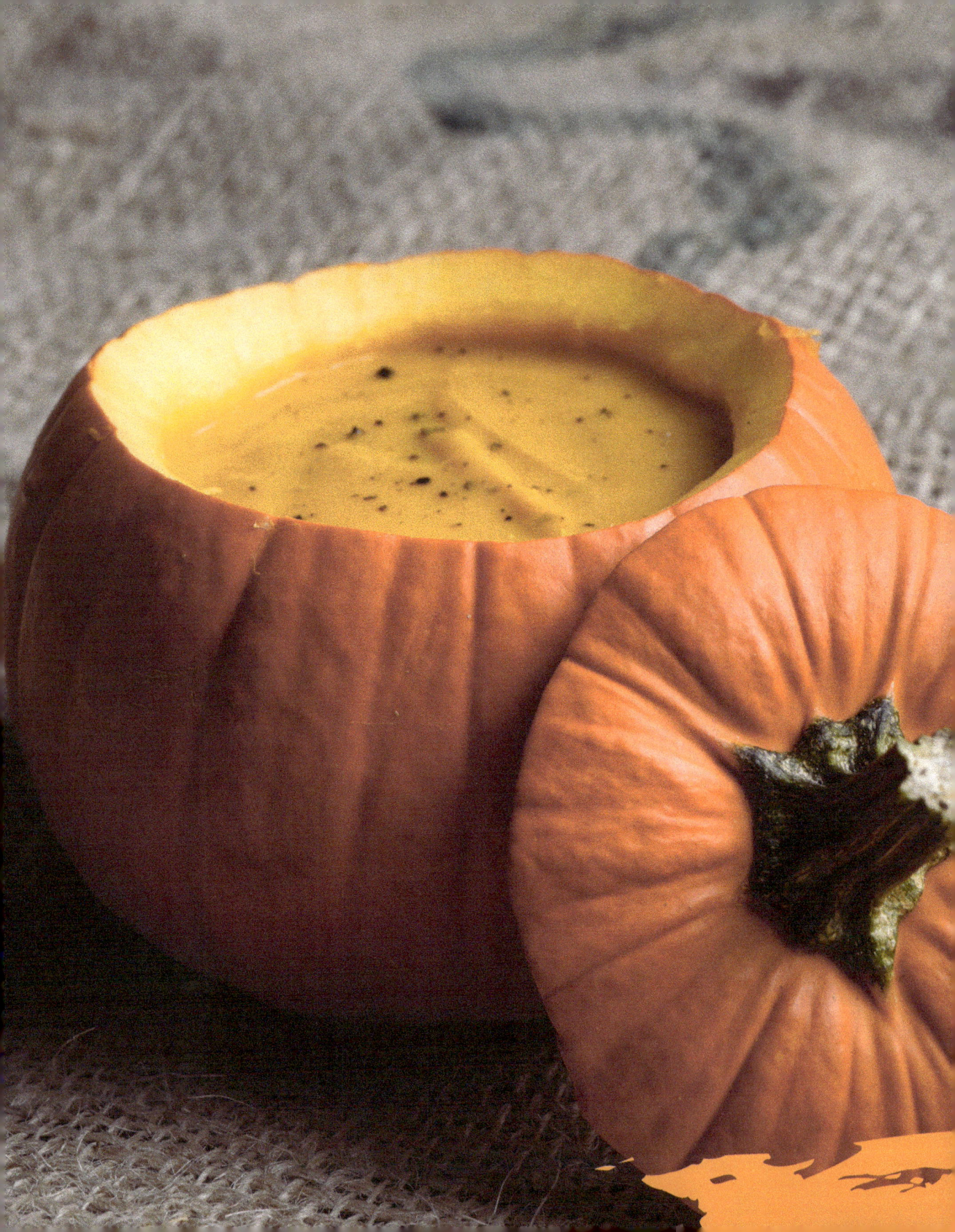

Sweet Pumpkin Soup

Kids' Favourite!

Serves 4

INGREDIENTS:

- 4 cups of mashed, roasted pumpkin. Sugar/pie pumpkins are especially nice (Butternut squash is also a good alternative). Depending on your variety, this can be made from about 4.5 lbs of raw pumpkin.
- 2-4 Tbsp organic maple syrup
- 1/3 cup olive oil, plus more to taste
- 2 tsp Celtic sea salt or Pink Himalayan salt
- Approx. 3 cups water, enough to liquefy your mashed roasted pumpkin in a blender
- 1 tsp flaxseed oil to drizzle on top (optional)
- A dash of pumpkin seeds, hempseeds, sunflower seeds
- A whole pumpkin, top cut off and insides cleaned out to serve soup in (optional)

DIRECTIONS:

Preheat the oven to 375 degrees. Wash and chop pumpkin into large pieces (skin on) and put them into a covered Dutch oven cooking pot. Pour in maple syrup, olive oil, sea salt and rub pieces of pumpkin well. Roast in the oven, covered, for 1 hour until pumpkin is soft. Separate the pulp, skin and seeds from the flesh. This roasted flesh makes up the base of the soup. Toss skin, seeds and pulp or eat them if you want to (I do!). Take the flesh and put it into a blender. Add water to just cover the flesh in the blender and blend on medium until it's creamy and it has reached your desired soup consistency. You may have to do several rounds in the blender as you go through all the pumpkin flesh. Put the creamy soup back into the Dutch oven and taste. Add more salt, maple syrup and olive oil as desired, and blend. Reheat on the stove and serve hot, topped with any pumpkin seeds or other seeds you may have, drizzle with flaxseed oil or olive oil. A fun idea is to serve it in a hollowed-out pumpkin for added smiles.

TRANSFORM

Cold Raw Summer Tomato Soup (Gazpacho)

Serves 4

Ingredients:

- 1 ½ pounds ripe tomatoes, chopped
- 3 cups of tomato juice
- 1 cucumber, chopped
- 2 red bell peppers, chopped
- 1 large red onion, chopped
- 1 small jalapeno, seeded and chopped
- 1 medium garlic clove, mashed
- ¼ cup extra-virgin olive oil, hempseed oil or flaxseed oil
- 2 Tbsp balsamic vinegar
- Juice of 1 lime or lemon
- 6 large basil leaves
- 1 tsp Celtic sea salt or Pink Himalayan salt
- ¼ tsp freshly ground black pepper
- 1 tsp smoked paprika (optional)

Directions:

This recipe is all about tomatoes and so the quality of the tomatoes you buy matters more than anything, as that will be the quality of your gazpacho. Be sure to buy nice, ripe, healthy looking tomatoes. Chop the tomatoes, cucumber, bell peppers, onions and jalapeno into chunks. Put those chopped vegetables into a big bowl and add in all of the rest of the ingredients. Take as much as you can at one time into your food processor or blender and blend until combined but not too smooth - you want to keep some chunks. Add water or a bit more tomato juice if needed to achieve your desired consistency. Combine all of the blended gazpacho in a serving bowl or glass water jug and place in the fridge until ready to serve. It's best to let it chill overnight rather than serving immediately as the longer the gazpacho sits, the better the flavour becomes. Drizzle with olive oil and garnish with parsley when serving. Will last in the fridge for up to 3 days.

Aga's Fish Chowder

Serves 8

Ingredients:

- 2 lbs white fish, preferably a type of fish listed under "Best Choices" or "Good Alternatives" on the Monterey Bay Aquarium Seafood Watch Consumer Guide (See the Seafood section in Section 1 of this book)
- 16-18 cups of water
- 3 medium onions, chopped
- 6 cloves of garlic, sliced
- 3 Tbsp Italian spice mix (with marjoram)
- 2 Tbsp wakame seaweed, dried
- ¼ cup olive oil or grapeseed oil for frying, or more as needed
- 3-4 tsp of your favourite savoury fish spice (just not lemon pepper)
- A pinch of hot chili flakes
- 1-2 tsp Celtic sea salt or Pink Himalayan salt, to taste
- 1-2 tsp fresh cracked black pepper, to taste
- A splash of balsamic vinegar (approx. 3 Tbsp)

Directions:

Coat the bottom of a large soup pot with olive or grapeseed oil and add your favourite fish spice, Italian spice and salt. Sauté over medium heat until you release the aromas, approximately 30 seconds. Add chopped onions and sliced garlic cloves. Sauté until onions are translucent. Add fish filet and sauté with the spices for approximately 1-3 minutes. Pour 16-18 cups of water into your pot. Put it back on the stove, lower heat to medium or low. Add sea salt and black pepper to taste, then add wakame seaweed and hot chili pepper flakes. Boil approximately 1 hour. Spike with balsamic vinegar to taste. Serve hot. Store leftovers in the fridge. Freezes well.

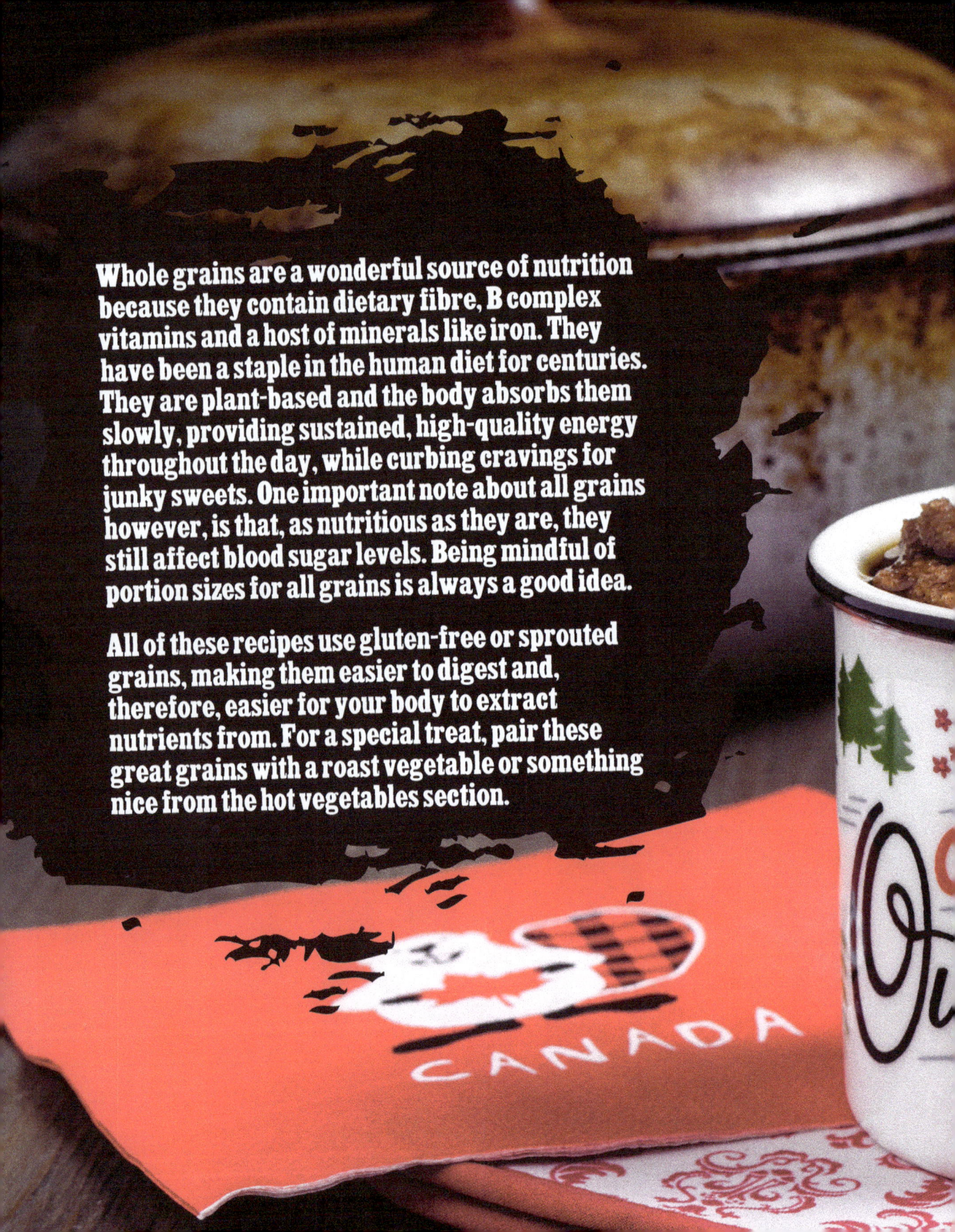

Whole grains are a wonderful source of nutrition because they contain dietary fibre, B complex vitamins and a host of minerals like iron. They have been a staple in the human diet for centuries. They are plant-based and the body absorbs them slowly, providing sustained, high-quality energy throughout the day, while curbing cravings for junky sweets. One important note about all grains however, is that, as nutritious as they are, they still affect blood sugar levels. Being mindful of portion sizes for all grains is always a good idea.

All of these recipes use gluten-free or sprouted grains, making them easier to digest and, therefore, easier for your body to extract nutrients from. For a special treat, pair these great grains with a roast vegetable or something nice from the hot vegetables section.

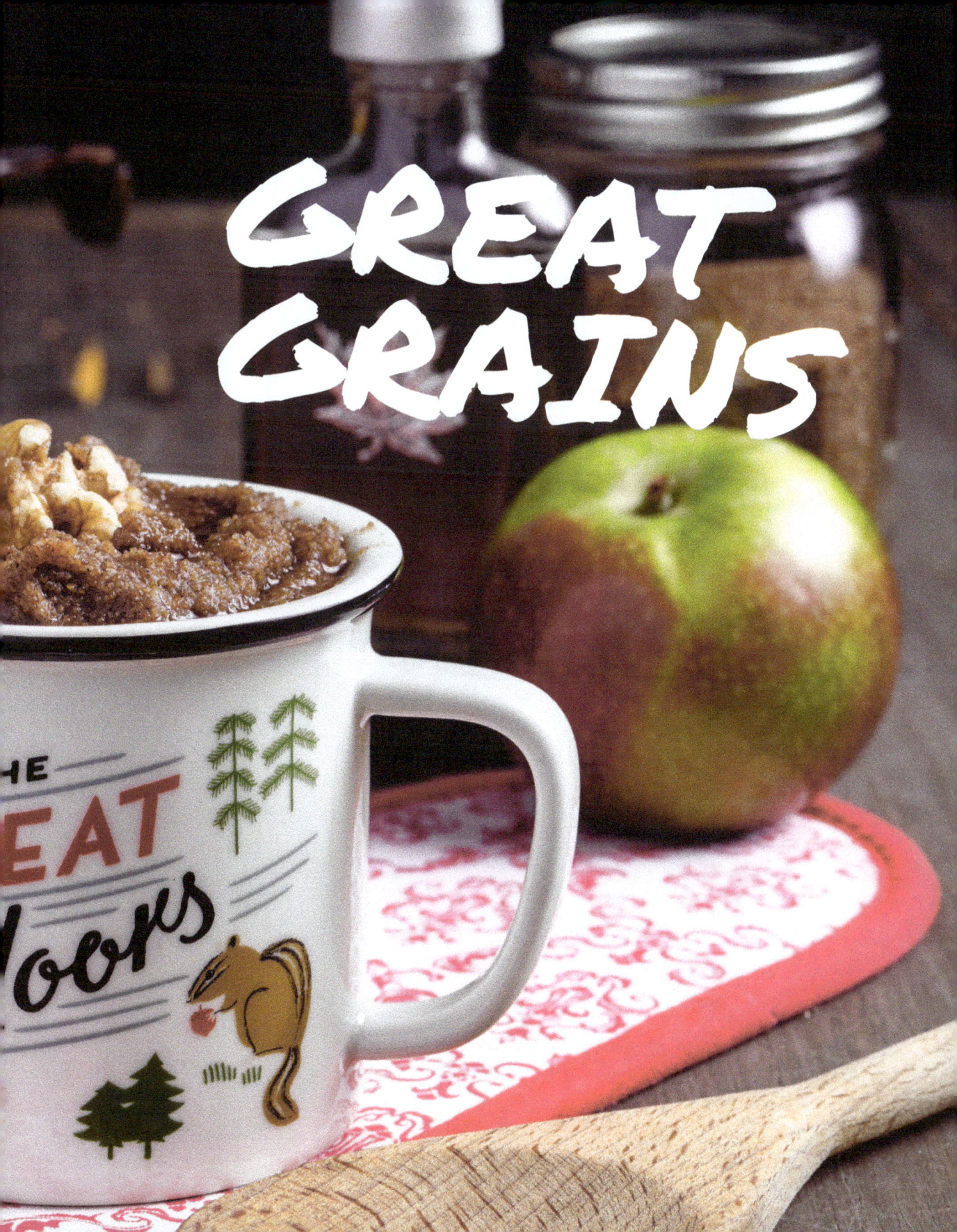

GREAT GRAINS

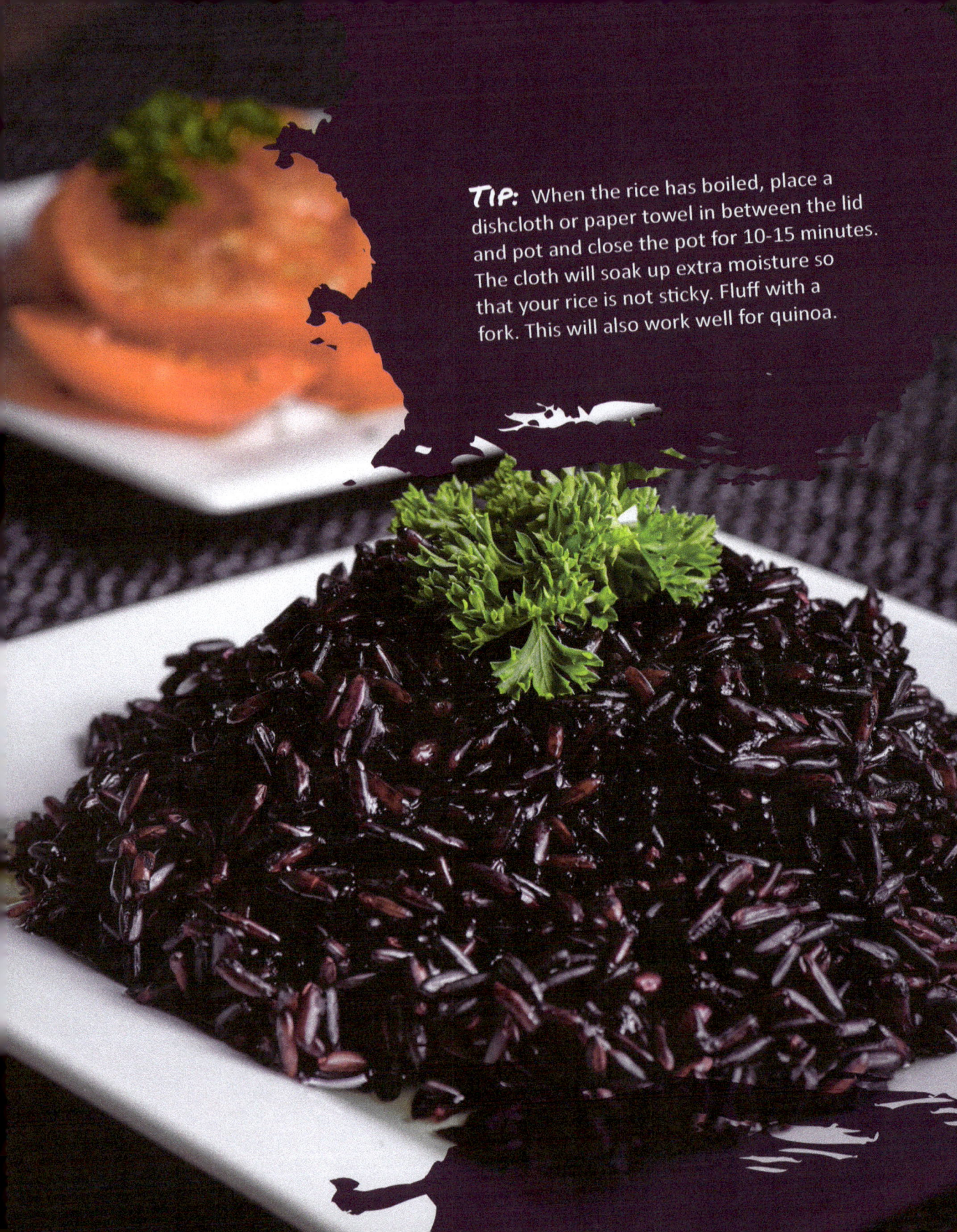

TIP: When the rice has boiled, place a dishcloth or paper towel in between the lid and pot and close the pot for 10-15 minutes. The cloth will soak up extra moisture so that your rice is not sticky. Fluff with a fork. This will also work well for quinoa.

Simple Forbidden Rice / Black Rice

Black Rice is the New Brown.

Serves 4

Ingredients:

- 1 cup black rice
- 1 1/2 cups water
- A couple pinches of Celtic sea salt or Pink Himalayan salt
- 1/4 cup Udo's Oil 3-6-9 Blend

Directions:

Rinse rice in water 2 to 3 times and drain. You can also soak it overnight in water for optimal digestion. Combine rice, water and sea salt in a saucepot. Cover and bring to a boil. Reduce heat to a simmer and continue to cook covered for 20-30 minutes or until all water has been absorbed. Remove from heat and let stand for 5 minutes covered, with a paper towel in between the lid and the pot to absorb excess water. Fluff with a fork. Serve hot with sea salt and drizzle Udo's oil over it. Store leftovers in the fridge. Double the recipe to have extra rice ready for other rice dishes throughout the week.

Savoury Turmeric Rice

Serves 4

Ingredients:

- 2 cups boiled rice (brown or basmati or black or whatever you have)
- 2-3 onions, sliced
- 1 garlic clove, sliced
- 2-3 Tbsp olive oil or grapeseed oil for frying
- 1 heaping tsp turmeric
- ½ tsp Celtic sea salt or Pink Himalayan salt
- Cracked black pepper to taste (optional)
- ½ bunch parsley, chopped (optional)

Directions:

Boil the rice and set aside.

Pour oil into a wok style pan or a regular frying pan and place over medium heat. Add turmeric and sauté until the flavours are enticed out of it, approximately 10 seconds. Add sliced onions and sliced garlic. Stir fry altogether. Add more oil so it glistens. Add sea salt and keep frying, mixing all ingredients around the pot until soft, golden, sweet and orange. Add rice and blend together on low heat until well combined. Add sea salt, cracked black pepper and parsley to taste. Remove from heat and serve hot to the ones you love. This works well with stir-fried vegetables. Store leftovers in the fridge.

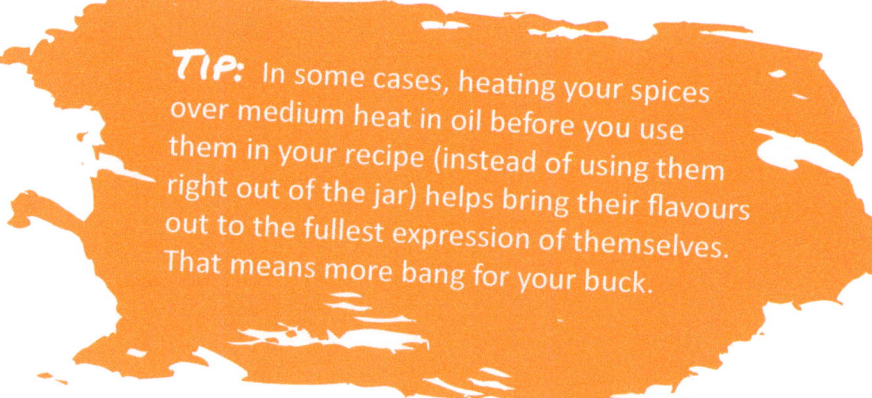

TIP: In some cases, heating your spices over medium heat in oil before you use them in your recipe (instead of using them right out of the jar) helps bring their flavours out to the fullest expression of themselves. That means more bang for your buck.

SPICY AND SWEET EXOTIC RICE

Serves 6-8

INGREDIENTS:

- 4 cups boiled rice (brown or basmati or whatever you have)
- 2-3 carrots, washed, peeled and grated
- 2-3 onions, peeled and sliced
- 4-5 garlic cloves, peeled and sliced
- ¼ cup olive oil or grapeseed oil for frying
- 5-6 oz of your favourite Middle Eastern spice mix (I like to use a Bermuda brand called Chiko's Smokey Rub – Middle Eastern)
- Approx. 2 Tbsp raw honey
- Pinch of Celtic sea salt or Pink Himalayan salt (if your Middle Eastern spice mix isn't salted)
- Pinch of ground cayenne pepper to taste

DIRECTIONS:

Boil the rice and set aside. Pour oil into a big soup pot and place over medium heat. Add 5-6 oz of your favourite Middle Eastern spice and sauté until the flavours are enticed out of it, approximately 30 seconds. Add sliced onions, sliced garlic cloves and grated carrots.

Stir fry vegetables with spices and oil. Add more oil so it glistens if necessary. Add sea salt and keep frying, mixing all ingredients around the pot until soft and golden sweet. Add rice and blend together on low heat. Add sea salt to taste. Add ground cayenne pepper to spice it up. Add honey to sweeten and to make it glisten even more. Some like it hot, but sweet too. Remove from heat and serve hot to the ones you love. Store leftovers in the fridge.

TRANSFORM

Quinoa Served Hot with Ginger, Garlic & Cilantro

Serves 4

Ingredients:

Plain Quinoa:
- 1 cup quinoa (experiment with varieties: white, red or black are the most commonly found although there are 120 known varieties!)
- 2 cups water

Dressing:
- 1 Tbsp fresh ginger, minced
- ¾ Tbsp Braggs Liquid Aminos
- ¼ cup brown rice vinegar (or whatever vinegar you have)
- 3 cloves garlic, peeled and pressed or minced
- ¼ cup fresh cilantro, chopped
- ¼ cup green onions, chopped
- ¼ cup toasted sesame oil

Directions:

Using a fine strainer, rinse quinoa with cool water. If you want to, you can toast the quinoa on a frying pan over medium heat for 1 minute before cooking to add a nutty taste (optional). Combine quinoa and water in a saucepan. Cover and bring to a boil. Reduce heat to a simmer and continue to cook covered for 15 minutes or until all water has been absorbed. Remove from heat and let stand for 5 minutes covered, with a paper towel in between the lid and the pot to absorb excess water. Fluff with a fork. In a large bowl, whisk all dressing ingredients together. Add cooked quinoa to your bowl and blend with the dressing. Serve immediately while still warm. You can add cooked, shelled edamame to this as well if you like. Store leftovers in the fridge, where it will stay fresh for up to 3 days.

Quinoa Salad (Cold Dish)

Serves 4

Ingredients:

Quinoa:
- 2 cup quinoa
- 4 cups water

Vegetables:
- ½ red onion, chopped finely
- 1 cucumber, diced
- 1 tomato, diced
- 1 bunch parsley or cilantro leaves, chopped
- 1 avocado, diced into cubes
- 1 cup edamame, shelled and cooked (optional)
- Simple Everyday Vinaigrette (See Sauces, Dressings and Spreads, page 203)

Directions:

Using a fine strainer, rinse quinoa with cool water. If you want to, you can toast the quinoa on a frying pan over medium heat for 1 minute before cooking to add a nutty taste (optional). Combine quinoa and water in a saucepan. Cover and bring to a boil. Reduce heat to a simmer and continue to cook covered for 15 minutes or until all water has been absorbed. Remove from heat and let stand, covered, until cool. Keep a paper towel in between the lid and the pot to absorb excess water. Fluff with a fork when cool. In a large bowl, whisk all dressing ingredients together. Add chopped vegetables. Add (cooled) cooked quinoa to your bowl and blend with the dressing and vegetables and serve. Store leftovers in the fridge, where it will stay fresh for up to 3 days.

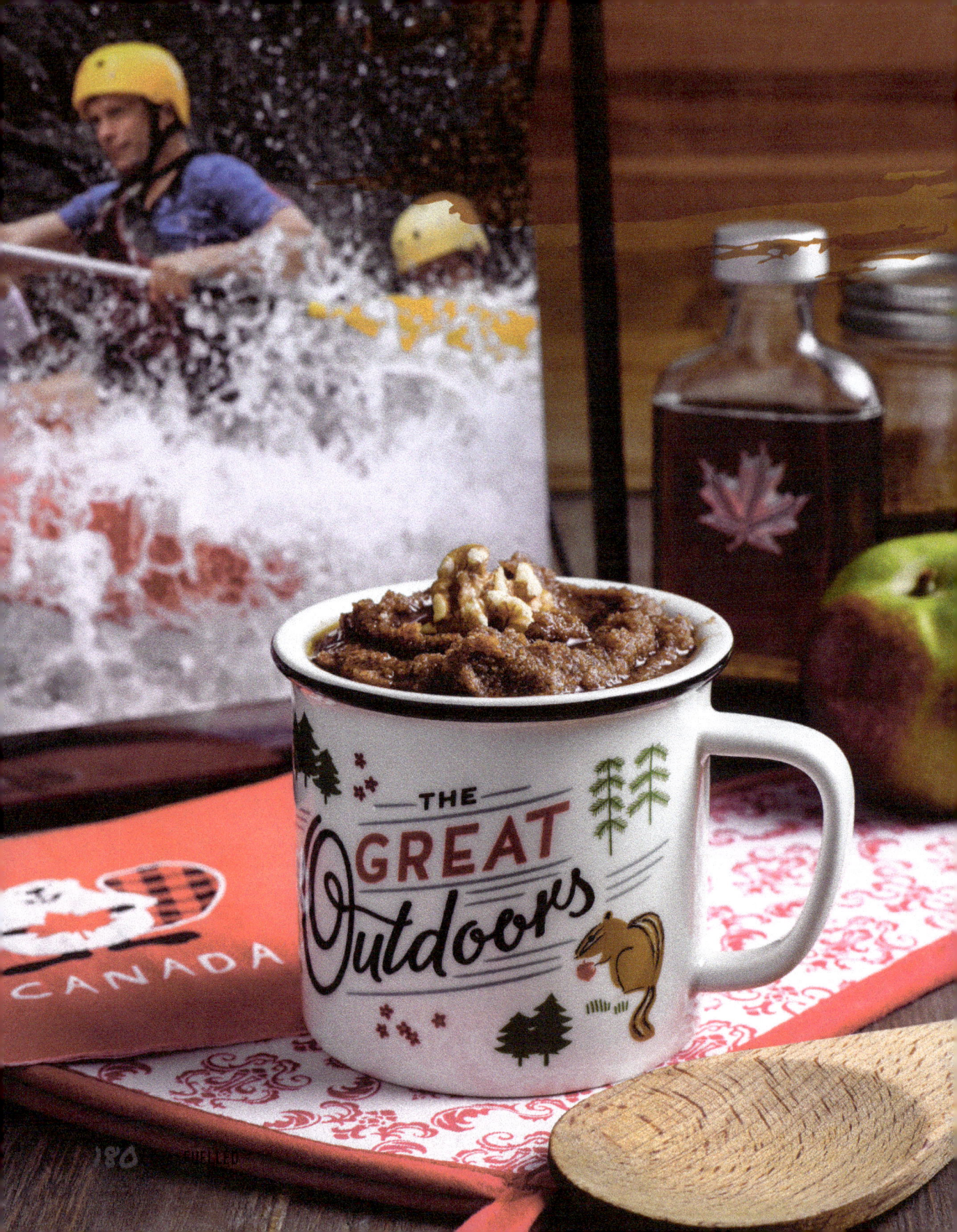

The Best Ever Teff Porridge

Kids' Favourite!

Serves 4

Ingredients:

- 1 cup whole grain Teff
- 3 cups water
- ¼ tsp Celtic sea salt or Pink Himalayan salt
- 2 tsp cinnamon, or more to taste
- 1 Tbsp extra virgin olive oil
- ¾ cup pitted medjool dates
- 2-3 Tbsp organic maple syrup, or more to taste
- ¼ cup walnut pieces
- ½ cup sliced and diced apple pieces
- ¼ cup non-dairy milk (almond milk, flaxmilk, etc.)

Directions:

Turn the stove on to medium heat and place a heavy Dutch oven on top of it. Heat the Dutch oven (dry) until it feels warm when your hand is close to it. Add teff and toast for 5 minutes, stirring frequently. It will make a popping sound. Add water, olive oil, cinnamon and pinch of salt. Stir well and bring to a gentle boil. Reduce heat a bit, cover and continue to cook for 10 minutes, stirring frequently. Do not leave unattended. You will need to stand close by and stir often or it will cook unevenly and clump (not that I know this from experience, wink, wink). Your porridge will thicken. Add in chopped dates, apples, walnuts and maple syrup. Cover and cook for 10 more minutes until the teff is tender and the porridge is thick. On another burner, heat up the milk in a small pot. When the milk is warm, uncover your porridge and add it in, stirring to combine well. This should create the most beautiful and velvety consistency. Remove from heat and let stand for 5 minutes (covered) before serving it in bowls and topping with maple syrup, sliced apples and a dash of cinnamon, or just as it is. Store leftovers in the fridge, they will last up to 3 days.

Optional:

Switch it up by trying different flavours (variety is the spice of life, right?). I would recommend Maple Pumpkin Spice (with maple syrup, pumpkin puree and pumpkin pie spice), Peaches and Cream (with peaches, honey, vanilla and extra milk), Blueberry Vanilla (with blueberries, honey and vanilla), and Maple Banana Nut (with maple syrup, banana slices and walnuts).

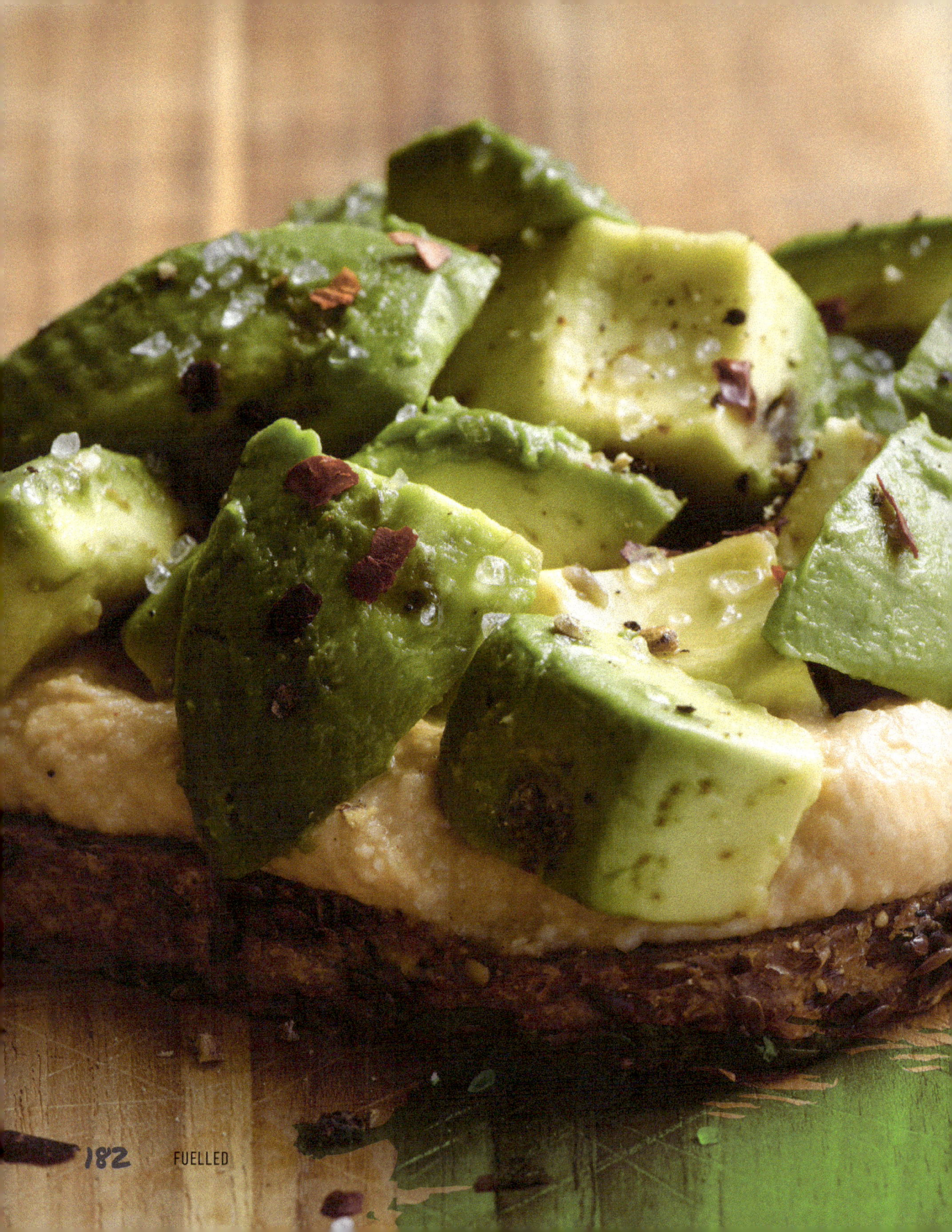

Avocado Toast on Fried Bread with Homemade Hummus

Kids' Favourite!

Yes, this is healthy folks.

Serves 1

Ingredients:

- 2 slices of Ezekiel or Genesis Brand sprouted grain bread
- 3 Tbsp olive oil or grapeseed oil for frying
- 1 ripe avocado
- A pinch of Celtic sea salt or Pink Himalayan salt, to taste
- A dash of cracked black pepper, to taste
- Homemade Hummus (See Sauces, Dressings and Spreads, page 199)

Directions:

First, make the hummus but putting all the ingredients in a blender or food processor until smooth. If it's too thick, add a couple tablespoons of water to thin it out a touch. Set aside. There is enough in this recipe to store in the fridge for a few days. Pour oil into a frying pan and place over medium heat. Take 2 slices of Ezekiel bread from the freezer and place (frozen) onto the hot pan. Fry for 20 seconds and then flip so that the other side is coated with oil too. Continue to fry both sides until they're golden on the edges and in the centre and nice and crispy on the outside. Smash the avocado using a fork or slice it up into pieces. Take a big tablespoon or two of homemade hummus and spread it on the toast, then top it off with the avocado. Sprinkle with sea salt and cracked black pepper to taste. Enjoy while toast is still hot!

TRANSFORM

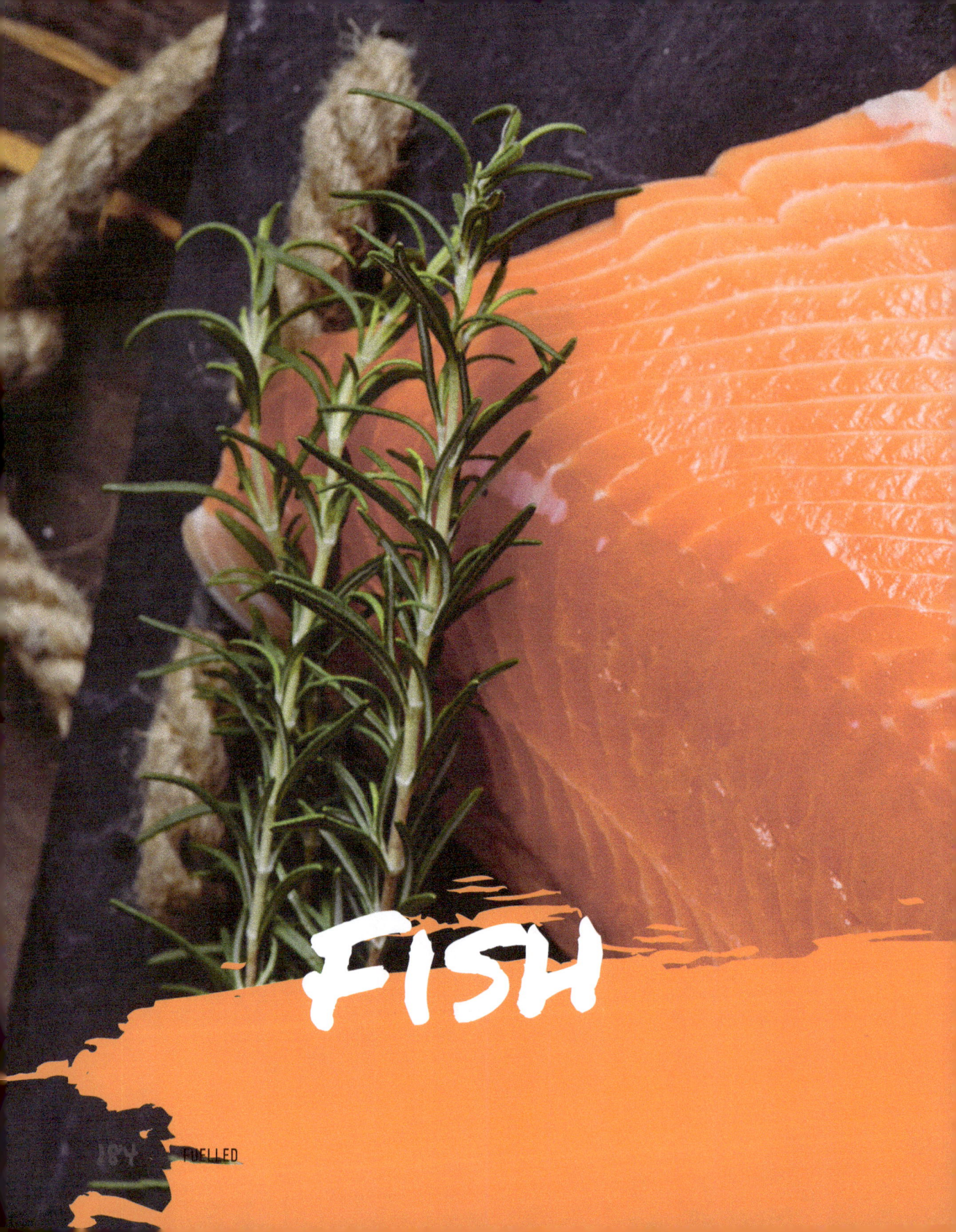

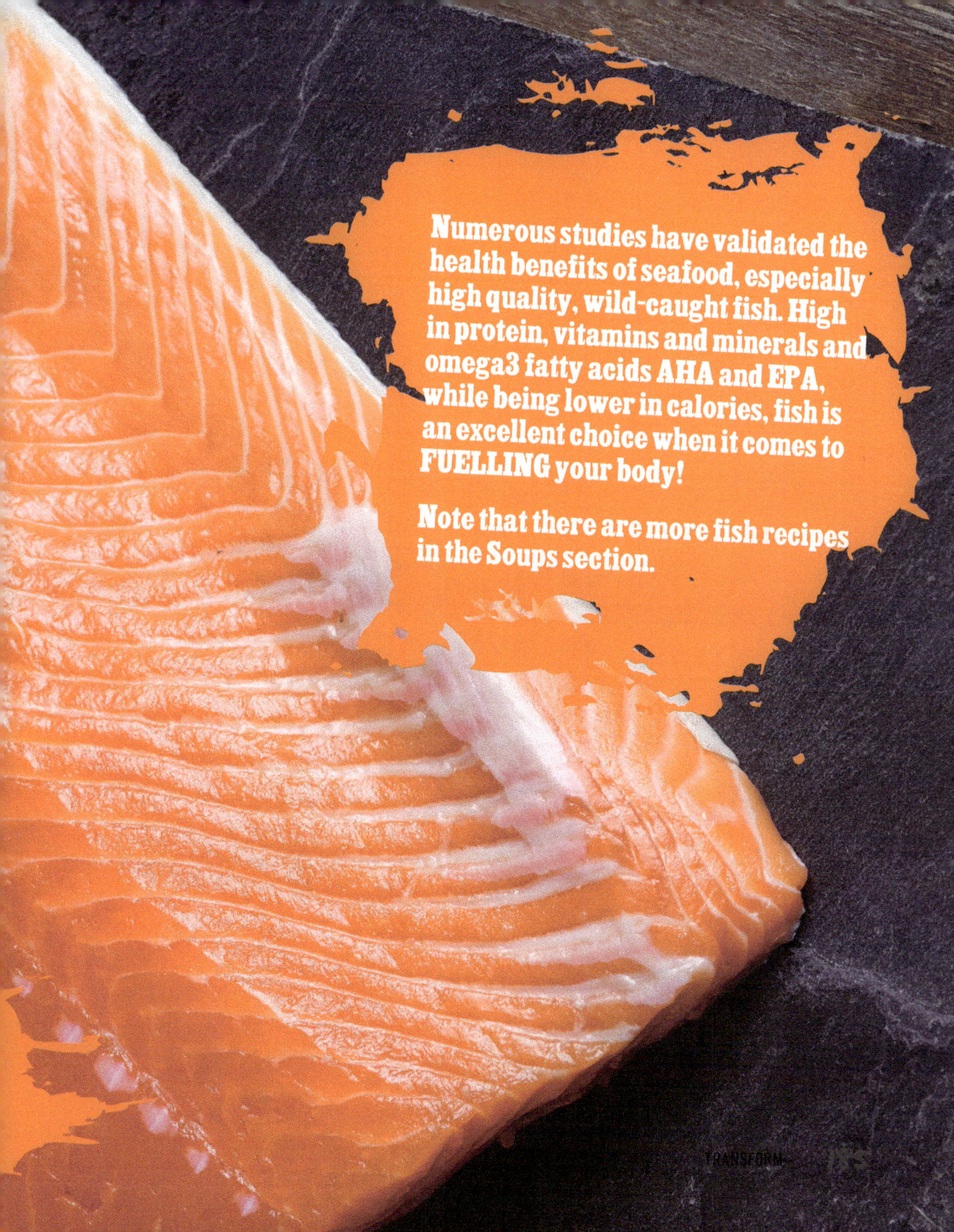

Numerous studies have validated the health benefits of seafood, especially high quality, wild-caught fish. High in protein, vitamins and minerals and omega3 fatty acids **AHA** and **EPA**, while being lower in calories, fish is an excellent choice when it comes to **FUELLING** your body!

Note that there are more fish recipes in the Soups section.

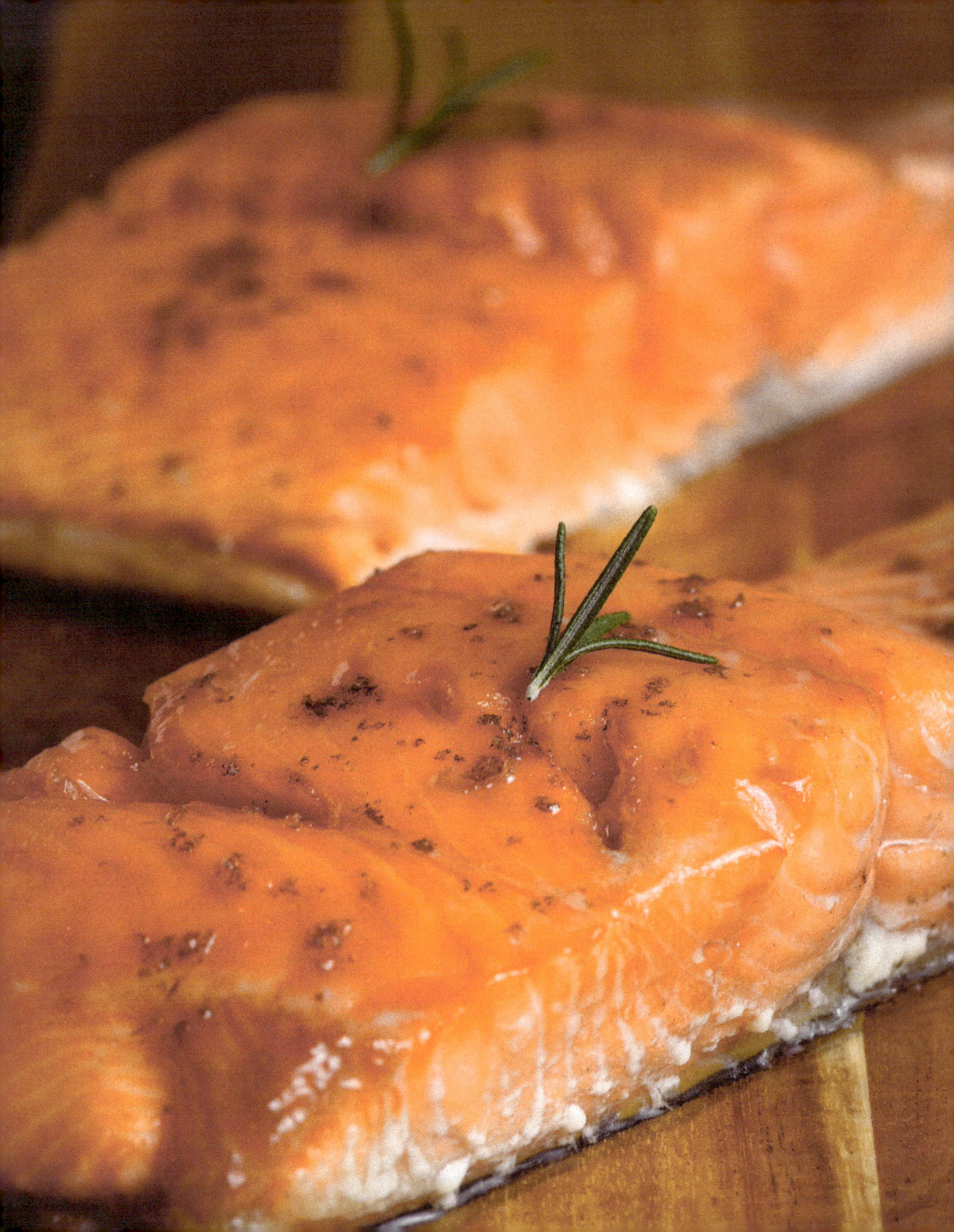

Smoked Salt & Maple Salmon

Kids' Favourite!

Serves 4

INGREDIENTS:

- 4 filets of Pacific Wild Caught Salmon
- 1 ½ tsp Alderwood Smoked Sea Salt (this is a specialty item that is worth finding online and ordering)
- 2 Tbsp extra virgin olive oil
- ¾ cup organic maple syrup

DIRECTIONS:

The day before you want to serve this salmon, put the oil, smoked salt and maple in a freezer size (large) resealable bag and massage the ingredients so that they combine nicely. Rinse salmon and pat dry with paper towels. Place the salmon into the marinade and seal the bag. Place it in a shallow dish and refrigerate overnight or for at least 4-6 hours. When ready to serve, preheat oven to 400 degrees, and remove salmon from fridge. Take the salmon and sauce out of the bag and place it on a baking dish. Bake for 10-12 minutes, depending on thickness, or until salmon is no longer raw in the centre but still very delicate and not tough at all. A little bit raw in the middle is totally okay with fresh, wild caught salmon. Again, I repeat, it should be soft and tender, melting in your mouth, not hard like a chicken breast. Remove from the oven and place your baking dish on the stovetop, or transfer the fish and sauce into a sauté pan. Sauté the fish in the maple sauce on medium heat for about 1-2 more minutes until the maple bubbles and thickens and the outside of the salmon is seared and darker in colour. Remove from the hot baking dish or sauté pan immediately so that the tender salmon stops cooking and place onto a platter, pouring the sauce on top. Serve immediately. Some people like to sprinkle crushed black pepper on top.

OPTIONAL:

You can switch up the flavour of the sauce (variety is the spice of life, right?) by using 2 Tbsp of Bragg's Liquid Aminos (a healthy soy sauce) instead of Alderwood Smoked Sea Salt and include 1 crushed garlic clove. That will make it a soy-maple glazed salmon. Very tasty. Sprinkle crushed black pepper on top or chopped green onions.

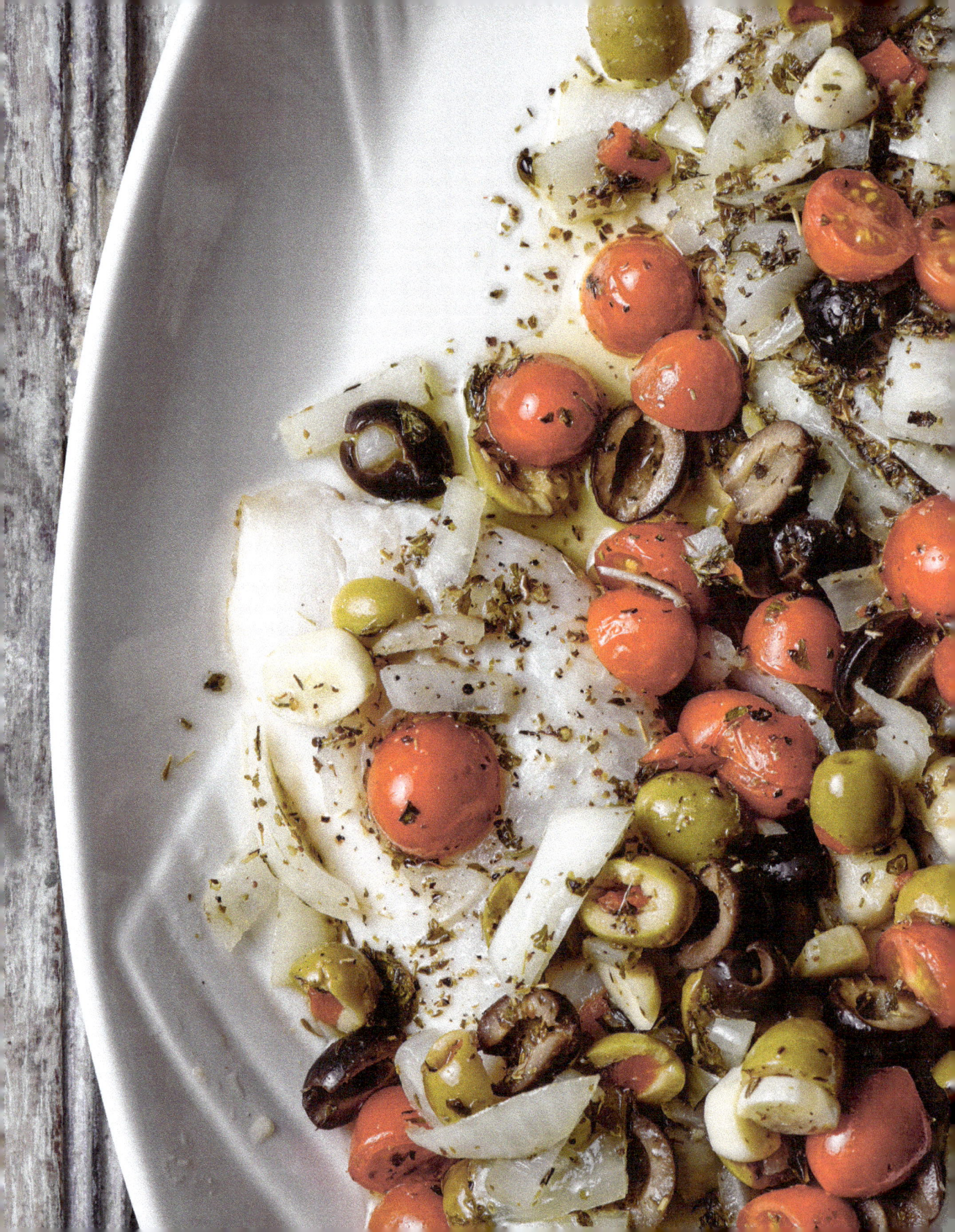

Baked Mediterranean White Fish

Kids' Favourite!

Serves 4

Ingredients:

- 2 lbs white fish, preferably a type of fish listed under "Best Choices" or "Good Alternatives" on the Monterey Bay Aquarium Seafood Watch Consumer Guide (See the Seafood section in Part 1: Educate of this book)
- ¼ cup extra virgin olive oil
- ½ cup olives, chopped
- 4 Roma Tomatoes, sliced in half, or 1 cup cherry tomatoes
- 2-3 cloves garlic, peeled and sliced
- Juice of 1 lemon
- 3 Tbsp dried oregano
- 1 Tbsp fresh or dried basil
- ½ tsp Celtic sea salt or Pink Himalayan salt
- 1 Tbsp dried parsley flakes

Directions:

Preheat oven to 400 degrees. In a bowl, mix together all of the ingredients except for fish. In a large wok or frying pan, sauté those ingredients over medium heat for about 5 minutes, until onions are translucent and garlic is cooked. Rinse the fish and pat dry with paper towels. Place the fish in a baking dish and pour the sauce on top. Using your hands, massage the sauce onto the fish. Bake for 12-14 minutes or until it is no longer raw in the centre but still very delicate and not tough at all. Again, I repeat, it should be soft and tender, melting in your mouth, not hard like a baked chicken breast. Remove from the hot baking dish immediately so it stops cooking and place onto a platter, pouring the sauce on top. Serve immediately.

Baked Wild Salmon with Cream Sauce

Kids' Favourite!

Serves 4

Ingredients:

- 4 filets of Pacific Wild Caught Salmon
- ½ cup of healthier mayonnaise* (make your own healthier mayonnaise with grapeseed oil or an olive oil/grapeseed mix** – see my recipe in Sauces, Dressings and Spreads, page 197) – or buy a vegan one that is not made with soybean, safflower, or canola oil - go for grapeseed oil if possible).
- 2-4 tsp of your favourite fish seasoning like lemon pepper, Cajun spice, garlic salt, a Caribbean fish seasoning, Italian fish seasoning, Polish fish seasoning (my favourite), etc.

Directions:

Preheat oven to 400 degrees. Rinse the fish and pat dry with paper towels. Place the fish in an oiled baking dish (so it doesn't stick). Take a heaping tablespoon of your mayonnaise and drop it onto one of your fillets. Smear it around so it covers the whole top surface. Do that to the rest of the fillets. Then take your favourite fish seasoning, sprinkle generously on the white mayonnaise and pop that into the oven. Bake for 12-14 minutes or until it is no longer raw in the centre but still very delicate and not tough at all. I repeat, it should be soft and tender, melting in your mouth, not hard like a baked chicken breast. Baked wild salmon that is a bit raw in the middle is what I prefer, to be honest, but cook it thoroughly if you prefer, as long as it's still tender. Take the salmon out of the oven and remove from the hot baking dish immediately so it stops cooking. Serve immediately.

*Okay, mayonnaise is not a health food but we all love mayonnaise and this recipe has made people who do not love fish, fall in love with salmon, and that matters.

** But do not make homemade mayonnaise with Udo's Oil 3-6-9 Blend *in this case* because this dish is going to be heated and you don't want to heat that oil.

Sardine Sandwich

This is an inexpensive, fast and easy way to enjoy fish protein and get your omega-3 essential oils in.

Serves 1-2

Ingredients:

- 3 cans of salt-free, wild caught sardines packed in water
- 1 to 2 tsp of your favourite fish spice – lemon pepper, Cajun, BBQ, or just a pinch of Celtic sea salt or Pink Himalayan salt and black pepper to taste
- 3 Tbsp olive oil, grapeseed oil or avocado oil, for frying

Directions:

Heat oil in a frying pan over medium heat until hot. Take the sardines, whole, out of the cans, discarding the water, and put them onto the hot frying pan. Sprinkle with your favourite spice. Fry up and mash into a paste on the pan with a fork (about 2 minutes). Remove from heat. Serve immediately on toasted sprouted grain bread. Enjoy!

Optional:

- Sauté with parsley, onions, garlic, sautéed together – they're all Superfoods!
- Sauté with olives
- Add tomato slices on top of your sandwich

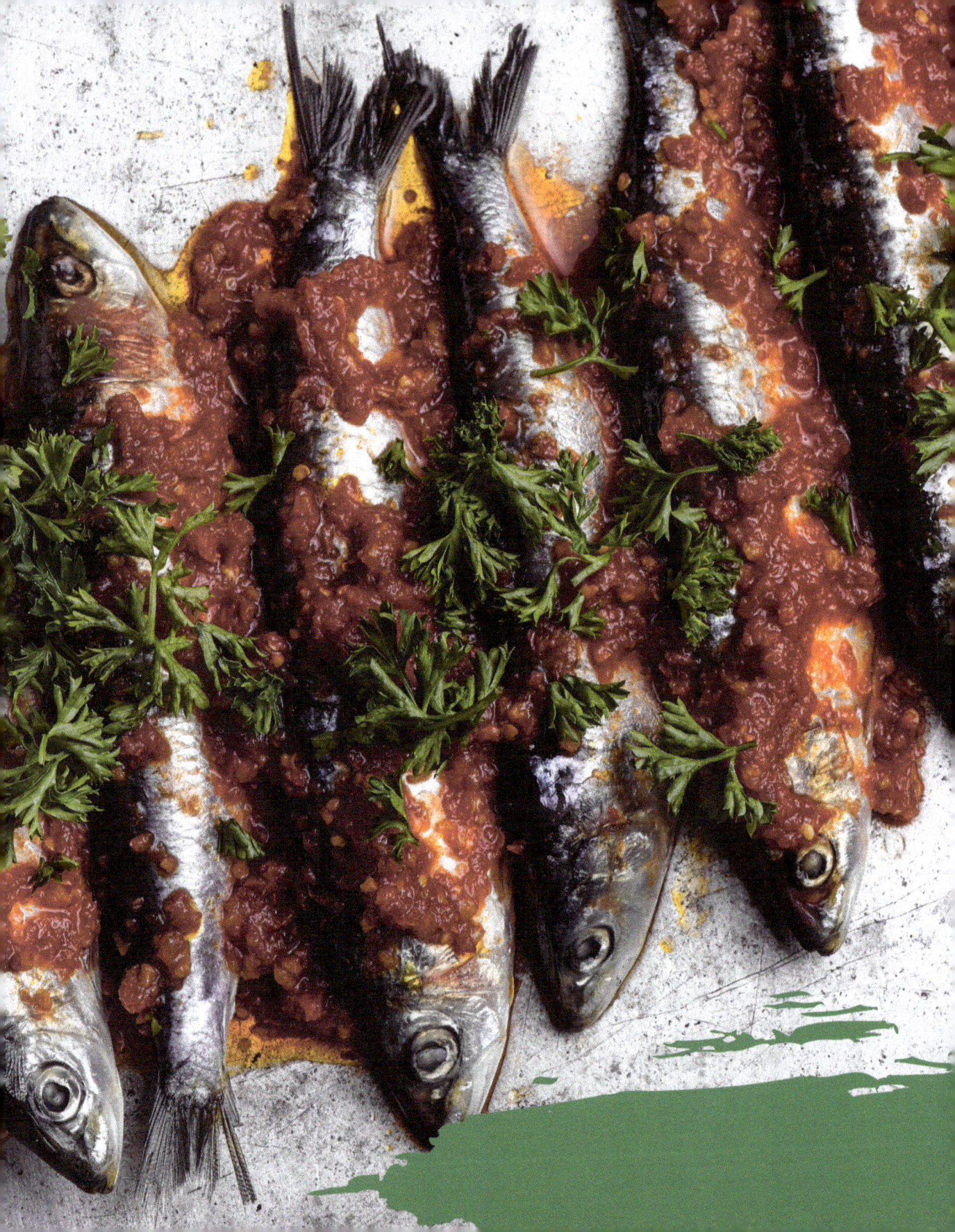

Easy Crushed Chili Baked Portuguese Sardines

Serves 4

Ingredients:

- 8 whole wild caught sardines (you can find these in most freezer sections of grocery stores)
- ½ cup crushed chili sauce, or garlic chili sauce
- ¼ cup extra virgin olive oil
- ½ tsp of cracked black pepper
- 1 Tbsp fresh parsley, chopped or dried parsley

Directions:

Preheat the oven to 400 degrees. If you bought the sardines frozen, what you want to do is to thaw them out in the fridge first. When thawed, take them to the sink and, using a dull knife, remove the scales by running the knife blade along the skin starting from the tailfin and moving towards the head. Keep the head and organs intact. Toss the scales out when finished and rinse off the fish. Pat the fish dry using paper towels, making sure they're as dry as possible. Place the fish onto a baking dish, rub with olive oil, pour on chili sauce and sprinkle with black pepper and parsley. Most chili sauces are already salted so salt may not be required at all. Place in the oven and bake for 12 minutes. Remove from the hot baking dish immediately so it stops cooking and place onto a platter, pouring the sauce on top. Serve immediately. They're a bit of work to eat, getting around all the small bones, but they're very tasty, and I like how the work causes you to slow down and chew properly, as you should, but often forget to do. Sardines are also great on the grill and you can try this recipe with grilled sardines, in which case I would sauté the sauce separately so it's hot and the flavours combine and the aromas are released, and then pour the sauce over the grilled fish.

SAUCES, DRESSINGS & SPREADS

Pictured: Aga's Fig Maple Vinaigrette, "Caesar" Salad Dressing, Omega Basil Pesto.

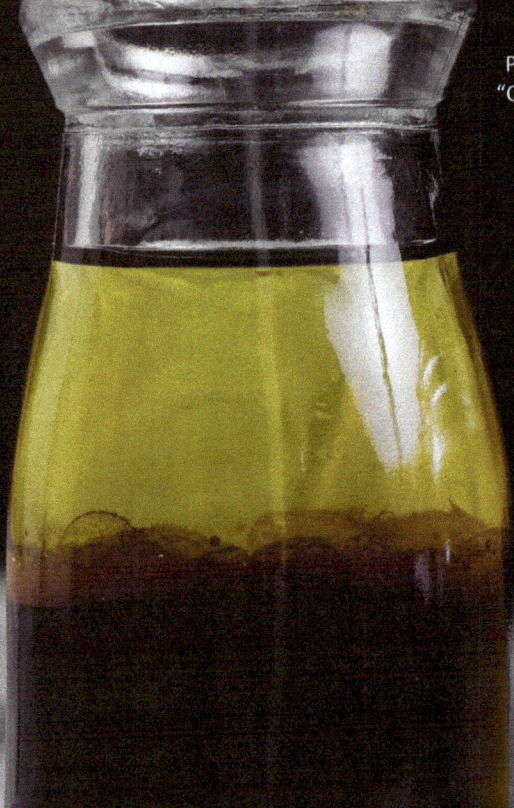

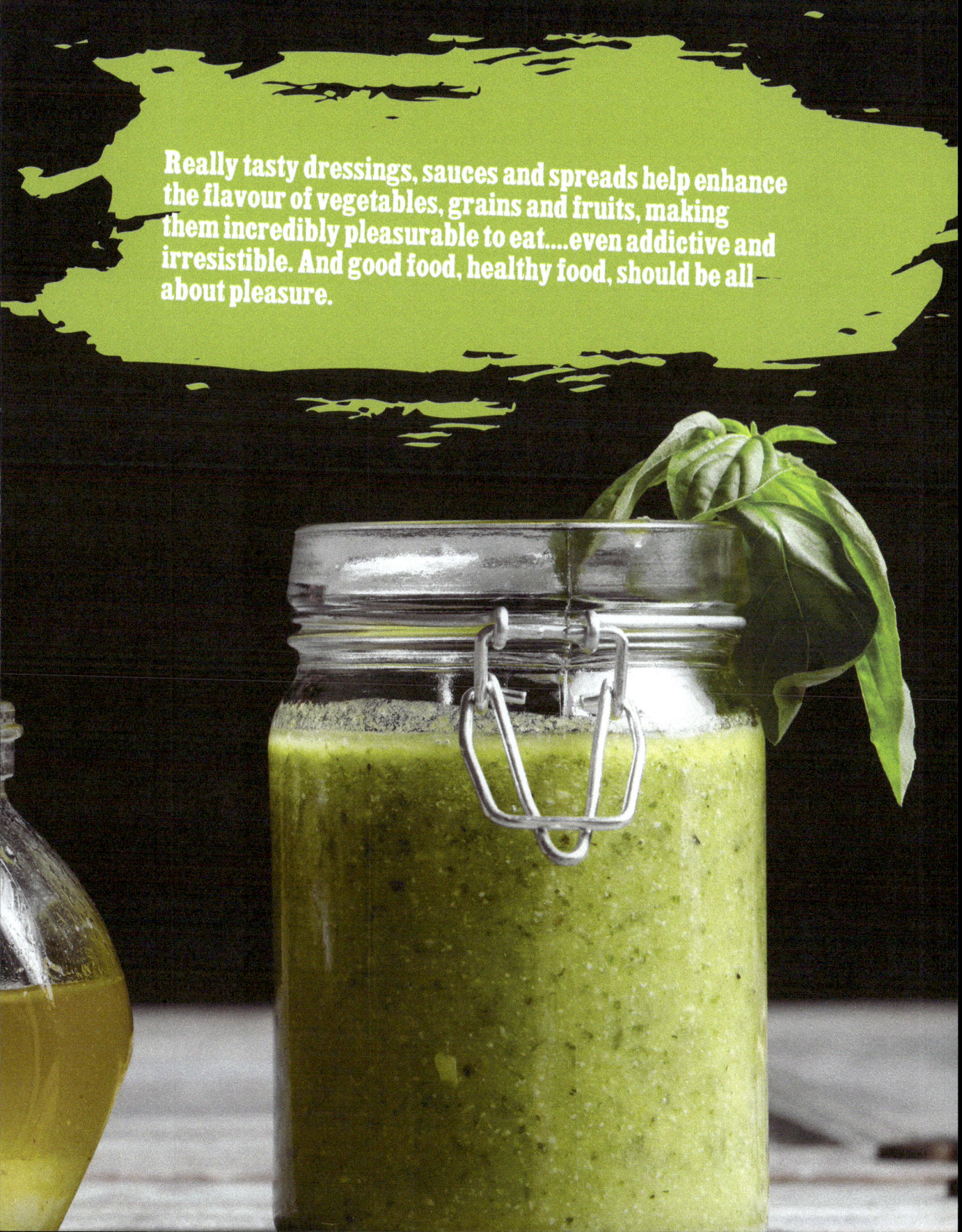

Really tasty dressings, sauces and spreads help enhance the flavour of vegetables, grains and fruits, making them incredibly pleasurable to eat.....even addictive and irresistible. And good food, healthy food, should be all about pleasure.

Omega Basil Pesto

This is my ultimate healthy basil pesto. A twist on the classic, it provides a powerful omega 3 and 6 punch when you use hempseed oil or Udo's Oil. Use this over baby greens, tomatoes, pasta salad, as a dip, or drizzled on top of fish. Do not heat.

Ingredients:

- 2 cups fresh basil leaves
- 1-2 cloves garlic, peeled
- ¼ cup hempseeds
- Juice of 2 lemons
- 1 cup hempseed oil, Udo's Oil 3-6-9 Blend (or extra virgin olive oil if you don't have those)
- ½ tsp Celtic sea salt or Pink Himalayan salt, or more to taste
- ½ tsp fresh cracked black pepper

Directions:

Blend everything together in your blender or food processor until smooth and store in a sealed mason jar until ready to use. This will last in the fridge for up to 3 days.

HEALTHIER MAYONNAISE

Sure, mayo isn't, traditionally, a health food, but what if you use a healthy oil like Udo's Oil 3-6-9 blend? Then you get to enjoy your treat and load up on your daily omegas at the same time. Here's a recipe for homemade mayo that is much healthier than any other you might have tried. Have fun with it and use it as a dip for your favourite vegetables, as a spread on your favourite sandwiches and in your salad dressings. There are countless exciting flavour combinations you can create using this mayo as your base. Just note that if you'll be heating the mayo, like in my **Baked Wild Salmon with Cream Sauce** recipe, do not use Udo's Oil 3-6-9 Blend as it isn't meant to be heated.

INGREDIENTS:

- 1 cup grapeseed oil, Udo's Oil 3-6-9 Blend, or half Extra Virgin Olive Oil and half grapeseed oil (olive oil is too strong a flavour for most people, so use a light version or a mix of these two oils)
- 1 large egg
- ½ tsp mustard powder or cayenne
- ½ tsp Celtic sea salt or Pink Himalayan salt
- Juice of 1 lemon

DIRECTIONS:

The day before you want to make your mayonnaise, put your oil and a metal or glass bowl in the fridge. Mayonnaise only works well when the oil, egg and bowl are cold. When you're ready to make your mayo, put the egg, mustard powder, lemon juice, salt and ONLY ¼ cup of your cold oil into your chilled metal or glass bowl. Using an electric egg beater/hand mixer or electric coffee frother (but not a blender), blend those ingredients. Then you need someone to help you hold the bowl, so grab a buddy. The next step is to very, very, very slowly, drizzle in the remaining oil, while blending it in with the other ingredients. I mean it: Slowly. In a thin stream. Your mayo will be thicker and creamier and less like soup the slower the remaining ¾ cup of oil gets blended in. When your mayo is ready, put it in a glass mason jar, seal it up and refrigerate immediately.

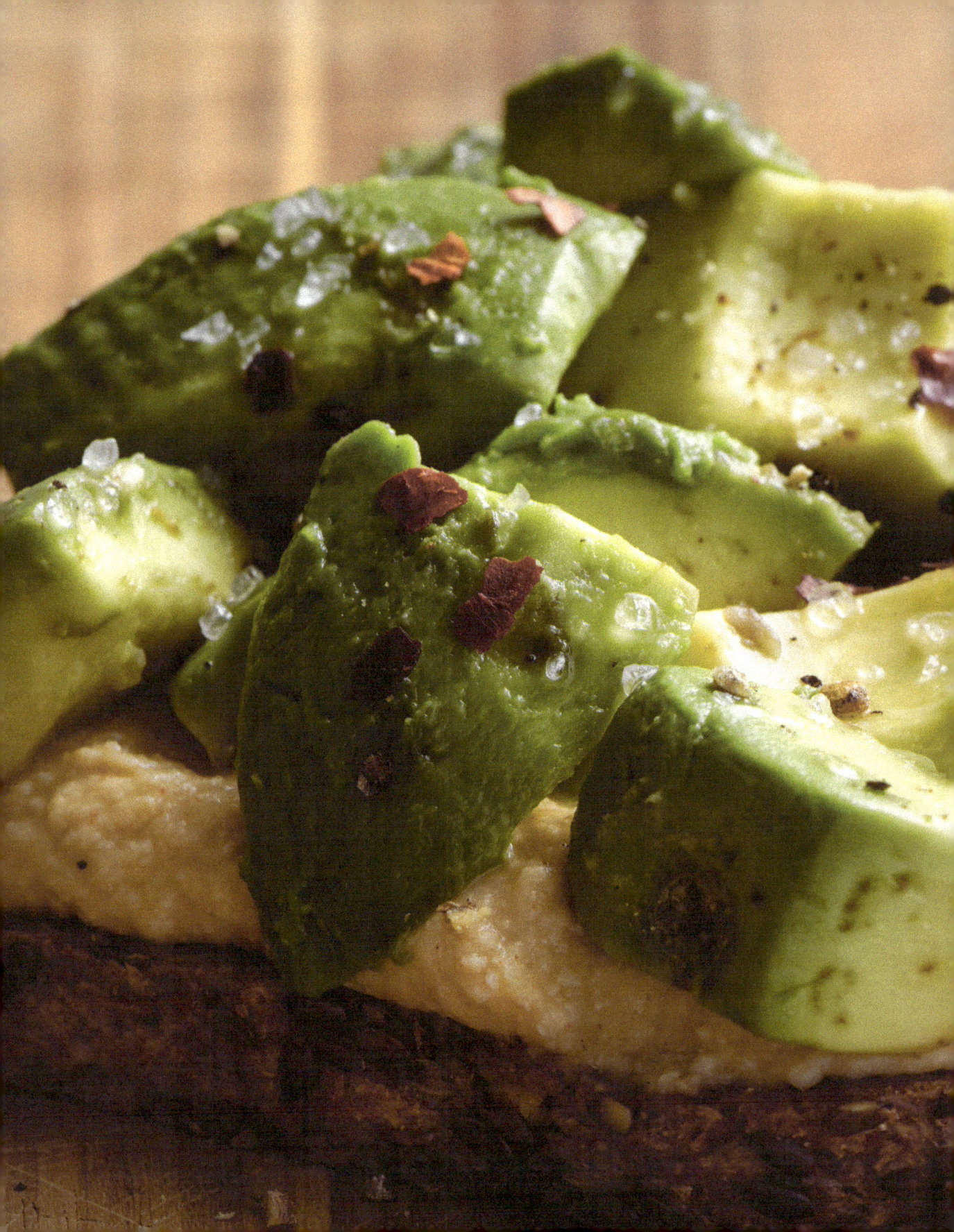

Homemade Hummus

Ingredients:

- 1 15 oz can of chickpeas, rinsed
- 1 clove garlic
- ¼ cup extra virgin olive oil, plus more for serving
- Fresh lemon juice of ½ lemon
- 2 Tbsp tahini (sesame seed paste, optional)
- ¼ tsp Celtic sea salt or Pink Himalayan salt, or more to taste
- ¼ tsp paprika (optional)
- Water

Directions:

Put all of the ingredients in a blender or food processer until smooth. If it's too thick, add a few tablespoons of water to thin it out a touch. Store in a sealed mason jar or glass container until ready to use. This will last in the fridge for up to 3 days.

Exotic Roasted Vegetables Sauce

Pour this over vegetables that you're planning to roast, especially if you've combined several vegetables together like leeks, zucchini, onions and garlic, or eggplant, tomatoes, onions and garlic. It's my favourite sauce for roasting eggplant in particular. An ingredient note: Bragg's Liquid Aminos sounds exotic and unusual but is available in most grocery stores and is simply a healthier version of the soy sauce you all know and love (but made entirely without wheat, unlike most soy sauces).

Ingredients:

- 1 ½ cups extra virgin olive oil
- ¾ cup balsamic vinegar
- ¼ cup plus 2 Tbsp Braggs Liquid Aminos

Directions:

Mix all of the ingredients together in a cup or shake them all together (much more fun) in a sealed mason jar until ready to use. This will last in the fridge for up to 3 days.

Sweet Basil & Honey Salad Dressing

Kids' Favourite!

This tastes great on baby greens, tomatoes, pasta salad, grilled fish, and fruit. It's super simple to make and an incredible salad dressing for summer.

Ingredients:

- About 1/3 cup or 20 larger leaves of fresh basil
- ¼ small onion, chopped
- ¼ cup light-coloured wine vinegar or apple cider vinegar
- ½ cup extra virgin olive oil, hempseed oil or Udo's Oil 3-6-9 Blend
- Juice of half a lemon
- 2 Tbsp raw honey
- ½ tsp Celtic sea salt or Pink Himalayan salt
- ½ tsp fresh cracked black pepper

Directions:

Blend everything together in your blender or food processor until smooth and store in a sealed mason jar until ready to use. This will last in the fridge for up to 3 days.

Pineapple & Pepper Salad Dressing

This dressing tastes great over mixed baby greens, fruit salads, goat cheese and walnuts.

Ingredients:

- 1 cup fresh pineapple chunks
- 1 orange, peeled and cut into chunks (or more pineapple)
- ½ cup pineapple juice
- Juice of 1 lemon or lime
- 1 Tbsp raw, organic honey
- 1 Tbsp apple cider vinegar or any other vinegar you have
- ½ cup hempseed oil, flaxseed oil, Udo's Oil 3-6-9 Blend or extra virgin olive oil
- ½ tsp Celtic sea salt or Pink Himalayan salt
- ½ tsp fresh cracked black pepper, or more to taste (I prefer more)

Directions:

Blend everything together in your blender or food processor until smooth and store in a sealed mason jar until ready to use. This will last in the fridge for up to 3 days.

Simple Everyday Vinaigrette

This is great on quinoa salad, greens, roasted vegetables or tomatoes.

Ingredients:

- ¼ cup apple cider vinegar
- ¾ cup extra virgin olive oil
- ¼ cup freshly squeezed lemon or lime juice
- 1 Tbsp parsley or cilantro, chopped finely
- 1 garlic clove, chopped finely or mashed
- 2 Tbsp raw honey
- 1 Tbsp Dijon mustard
- ½ tsp Celtic sea salt or Pink Himalayan salt
- Pinch of cracked black pepper
- Pinch of cayenne pepper (optional)

Directions:

Mix all of the ingredients together in a cup or shake all together (much more fun) in a sealed mason jar. Store in a sealed mason jar until ready to use. This will last in the fridge for up to 3 days.

"Caesar" Salad Dressing

This is my mother's recipe (the olive oil version). Use over mixed greens, romaine lettuce, or it tastes especially nice over a blend of kale and baby spinach.

Ingredients:

- ½ cup extra virgin olive oil or Udo's Oil 3-6-9 Blend
- 2 garlic cloves, peeled and crushed
- Juice of 1 lemon
- ½ tsp Celtic sea salt or Pink Himalayan salt, or more to taste
- ½ tsp fresh cracked black pepper

Directions:

Mix all of the ingredients together in a cup or shake them all together (much more fun) in a sealed mason jar. Store in a sealed mason jar until ready to use. This will last in the fridge for up to 3 days.

Aga's Fig Maple Vinaigrette

Kids' Favourite!

This is my secret sauce!! It will turn anyone into a lover of baby spinach salad. Also amazing on fruit and soft goat cheese. It's the perfect salad dressing for Summer.

Ingredients:

- ½ cup hempseed oil (or olive or flaxseed if you have those on hand, or Udo's Oil 3-6-9 Blend, but hempseed is the best for this)
- ½ cup organic maple syrup
- 3 Tbsp fruity dark red vinegar like fig balsamic vinegar or cherry balsamic vinegar

Directions:

Mix all of the ingredients together in a cup or shake all together (much more fun) in a sealed mason jar. Store in a sealed mason jar until ready to use. This recipe makes enough for up to 3 salads, not just 1. It will last in the fridge for up to 5 days.

Aga's Apple Cider Vinaigrette

Kids' Favourite!

This is a lighter version of my secret sauce.

Ingredients:

- ½ cup hempseed oil (or olive or flaxseed if you have those on hand, but hempseed is the best for this)
- ½ cup organic maple syrup
- 3 Tbsp apple cider vinegar

Directions:

Mix all of the ingredients together in a cup or shake them all together (much more fun) in a sealed mason jar. Store in a sealed mason jar until ready to use. This recipe makes enough for up to 2 salads, not just 1. It will last in the fridge for up to 5 days.

TAHINI DRESSING

Don't be intimidated by tahini. It sounds exotic but it's just sesame seed butter. Think peanut butter, but made from sesame seeds. It tastes amazing when used as an ingredient in many recipes. This dressing is great on roasted vegetables, like cauliflower, or over baked white fish.

INGREDIENTS:

- ¾ cup organic tahini
- Juice of 2 lemons
- 2 garlic cloves, mashed
- 3 Tbsp extra virgin olive oil, hempseed oil or Udos Oil
- 2 tsp sea salt
- ¼ cup fresh parsley, finely chopped
- water

DIRECTIONS:

Mix all of the ingredients together in a bowl, except for water. Then slowly add enough water to make a thick sauce. Store in a sealed mason jar until ready to use. This will last in the fridge for up to 3 days.

Tahini Dressing – Sweet

Kids' Favourite!

This tastes great on sweeter salads, like ones that feature fruit.

Ingredients:

- ½ cup organic tahini
- 2 Tbsp extra virgin olive oil, hempseed oil or Udos Oil
- 2 tsp organic maple syrup
- 1 Tbsp fresh organic lemon juice
- water

Directions:

Mix all of the ingredients together in a bowl, except for water. Then slowly add enough water to make a thick sauce. Store in a sealed mason jar until ready to use. This will last in the fridge for up to 3 days.

Super Fun Chia Berry Jam

Kids' Favourite!

You might have seen chia jam in the grocery store, this is a delicious and simple way to make your own. Kids love this recipe!

Ingredients:

- 3 cups of raspberries, blackberries, strawberries, pitted cherries or blueberries (fresh or frozen but thawed)
- 4 Tbsp raw honey
- 2-3 Tbsp chia seeds
- 1 tsp raw vanilla bean powder

Directions:

In a bowl, combine your berries and honey and mash them gently. Then place this berry mash onto a non-stick frying pan and bring to a simmer over medium heat, stirring frequently. This takes about 5 minutes. Pour in the chia seeds and blend thoroughly. Continue to heat for about 15 more minutes, stirring frequently, until the mixture thickens. Add the vanilla bean powder in at the end. Remove from heat and let cool. It will thicken even more as it cools. Store in a sealed mason jar until ready to use. This will last in the fridge for 5-10 days.

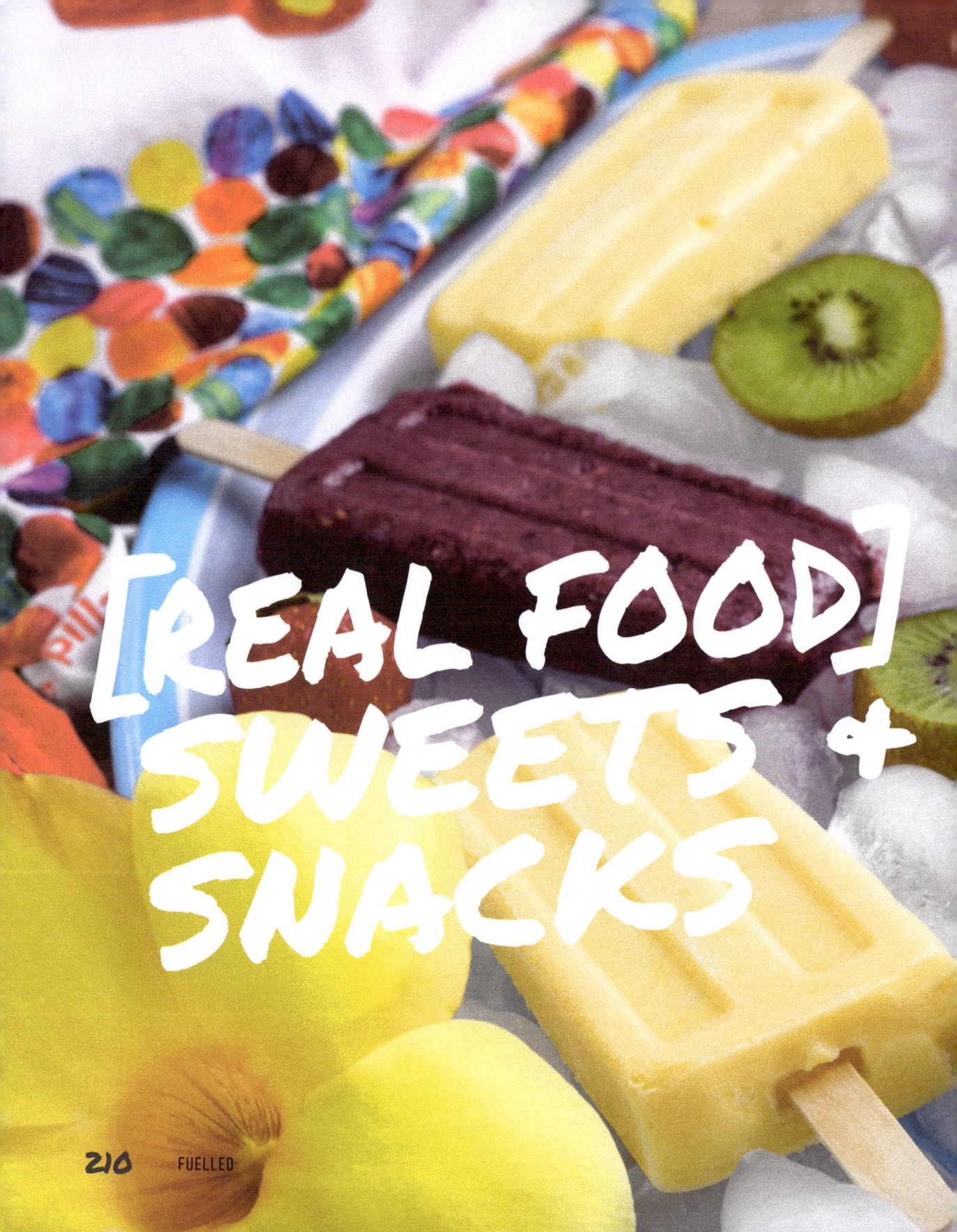

[REAL FOOD] SWEETS & SNACKS

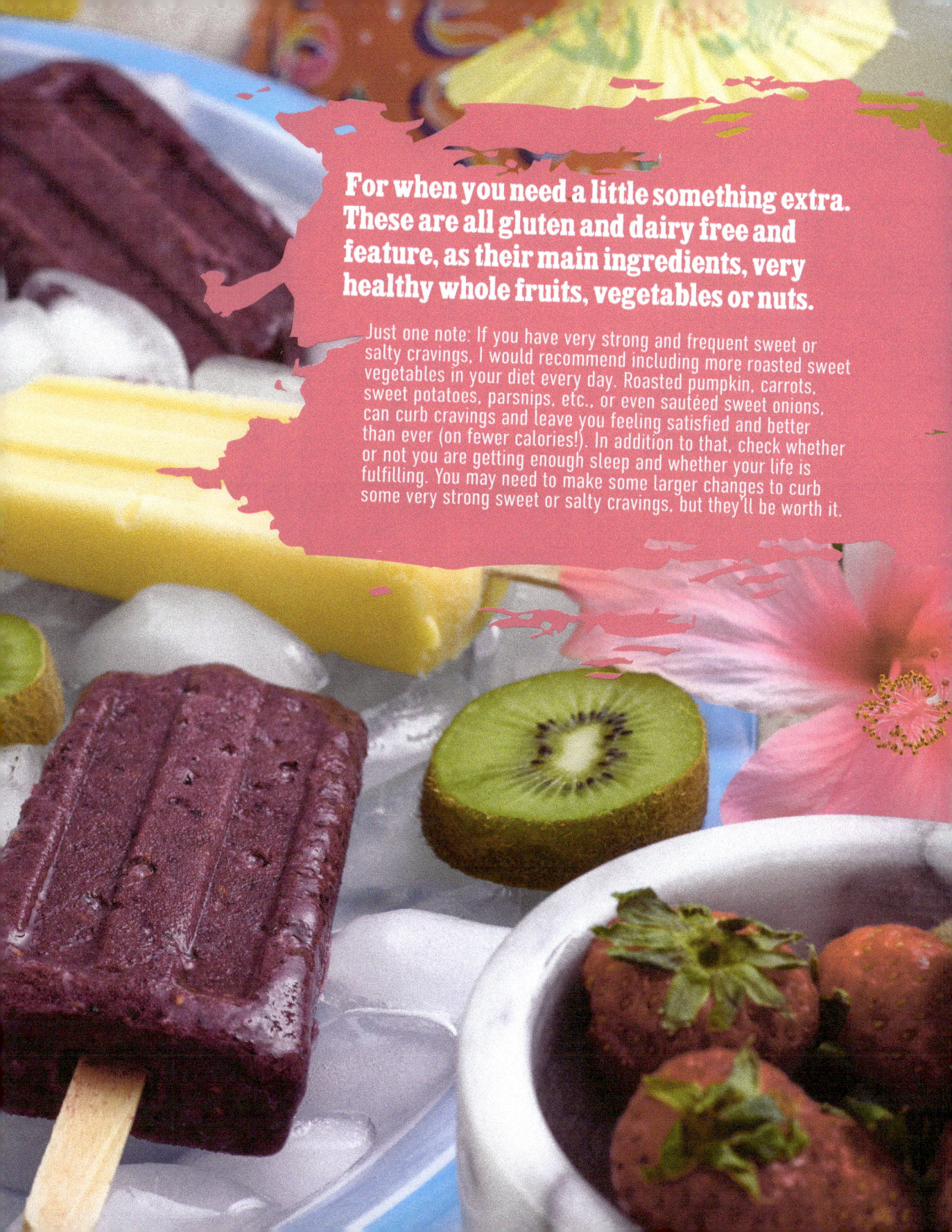

For when you need a little something extra. These are all gluten and dairy free and feature, as their main ingredients, very healthy whole fruits, vegetables or nuts.

Just one note: If you have very strong and frequent sweet or salty cravings, I would recommend including more roasted sweet vegetables in your diet every day. Roasted pumpkin, carrots, sweet potatoes, parsnips, etc., or even sautéed sweet onions, can curb cravings and leave you feeling satisfied and better than ever (on fewer calories!). In addition to that, check whether or not you are getting enough sleep and whether your life is fulfilling. You may need to make some larger changes to curb some very strong sweet or salty cravings, but they'll be worth it.

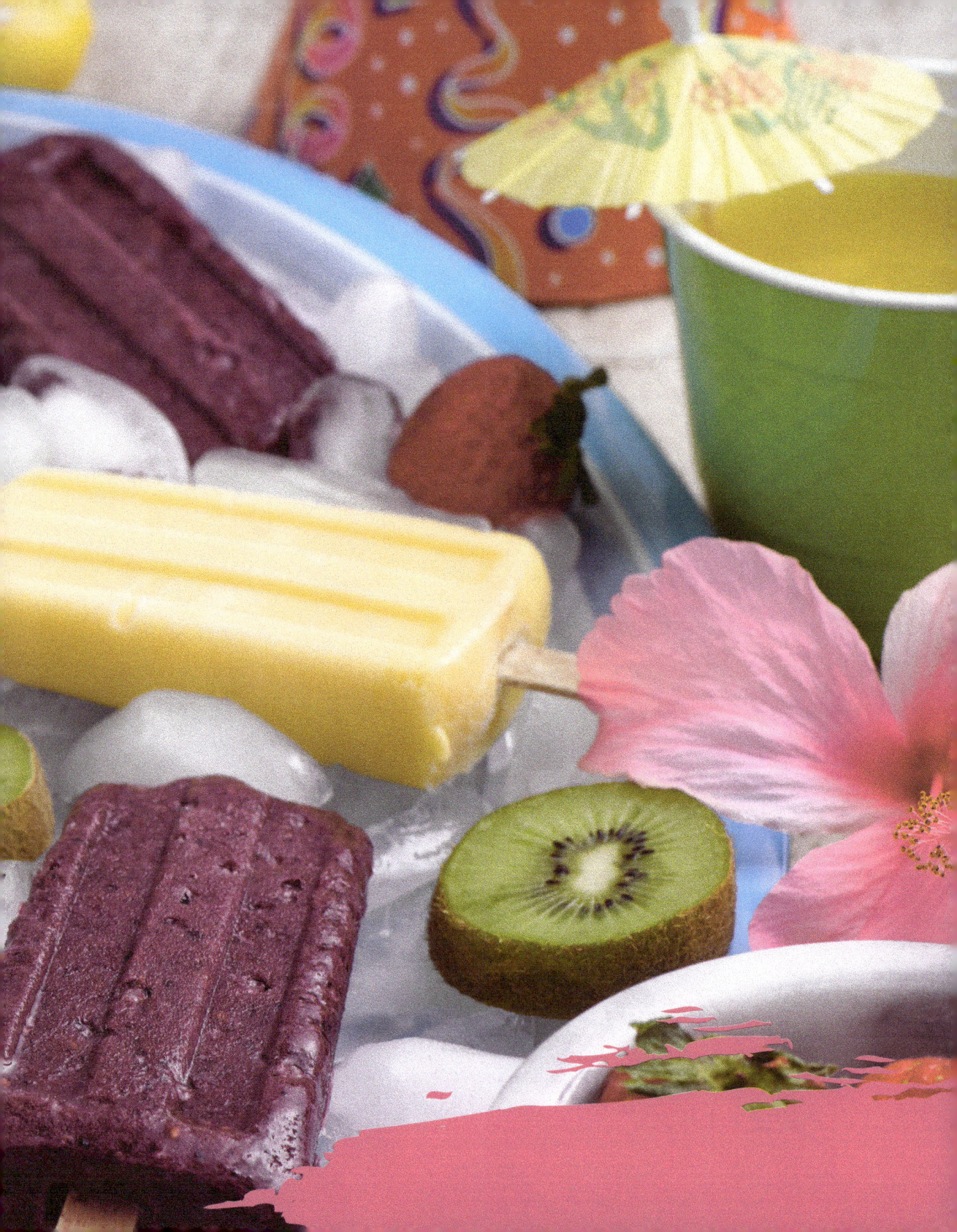

SUMMERTIME POPSICLES

Kids' Favourite!

This is an easy-peasy dessert that is fun for kids and adults alike. To make summertime popsicles, combine all the ingredients in a blender and blend until smooth. Pour the mixture into popsicle moulds, insert popsicles sticks, and freeze until solid.

makes 10 popsicles

INGREDIENTS:

Mango:
- 3 cups mango (fresh or frozen)
- 1 banana
- 7-8 Tbsp full fat coconut milk
- 2 Tbsp raw honey

Berry:
- 3 cups strawberries, raspberries, blueberries, blackberries (fresh or frozen)
- 1 banana
- 8 Tbsp pineapple juice
- 4 Tbsp raw honey

Aloha Awakening (Pineapple and Coconut):
- 1 can full fat coconut milk
- 1 cup of fresh pineapple (cut into small bits)
- 1 cup of mango chunks
- 1 banana
- 4 Tbsp raw honey

Maple Banana Nut Dream:
- 3 cups bananas, mashed
- 1 can of full fat coconut milk
- 3-4 Tbsp soy nut butter
- 2 Tbsp organic maple syrup

TRANSFORM

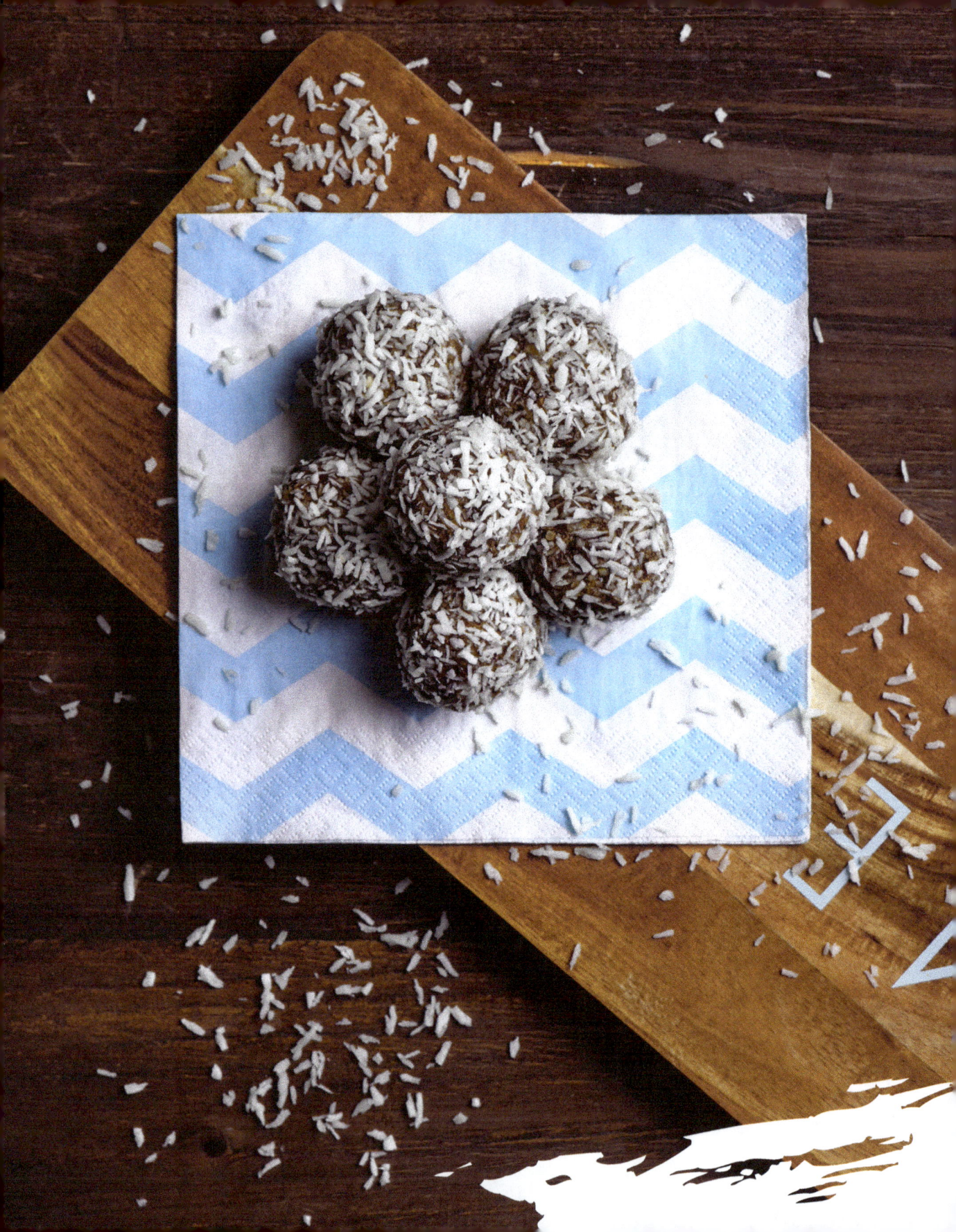

Walnut Coconut Balls

Kids' Favourite!

Serves 4

Ingredients:

- 1 cup pitted medjool dates
- 1½ cups walnuts
- ½ cup unsweetened coconut flakes
- 4 Tbsp virgin coconut oil
- 3 Tbsp hempseeds
- 1 tsp vanilla bean powder (or ½ teaspoon of vanilla extract)

Directions:

Combine walnuts and coconut oil in a blender or food processor and blend until the nuts are ground. Add dates and blend until sticky and smooth. Add hempseeds, vanilla bean powder and coconut flakes, blending until well combined. Roll into balls then roll the balls in a plate filled with more unsweetened coconut flakes and place into refrigerator for approximately 1 hour, until they're nice and firm, and then serve. Store leftovers in the fridge for up to 5 days.

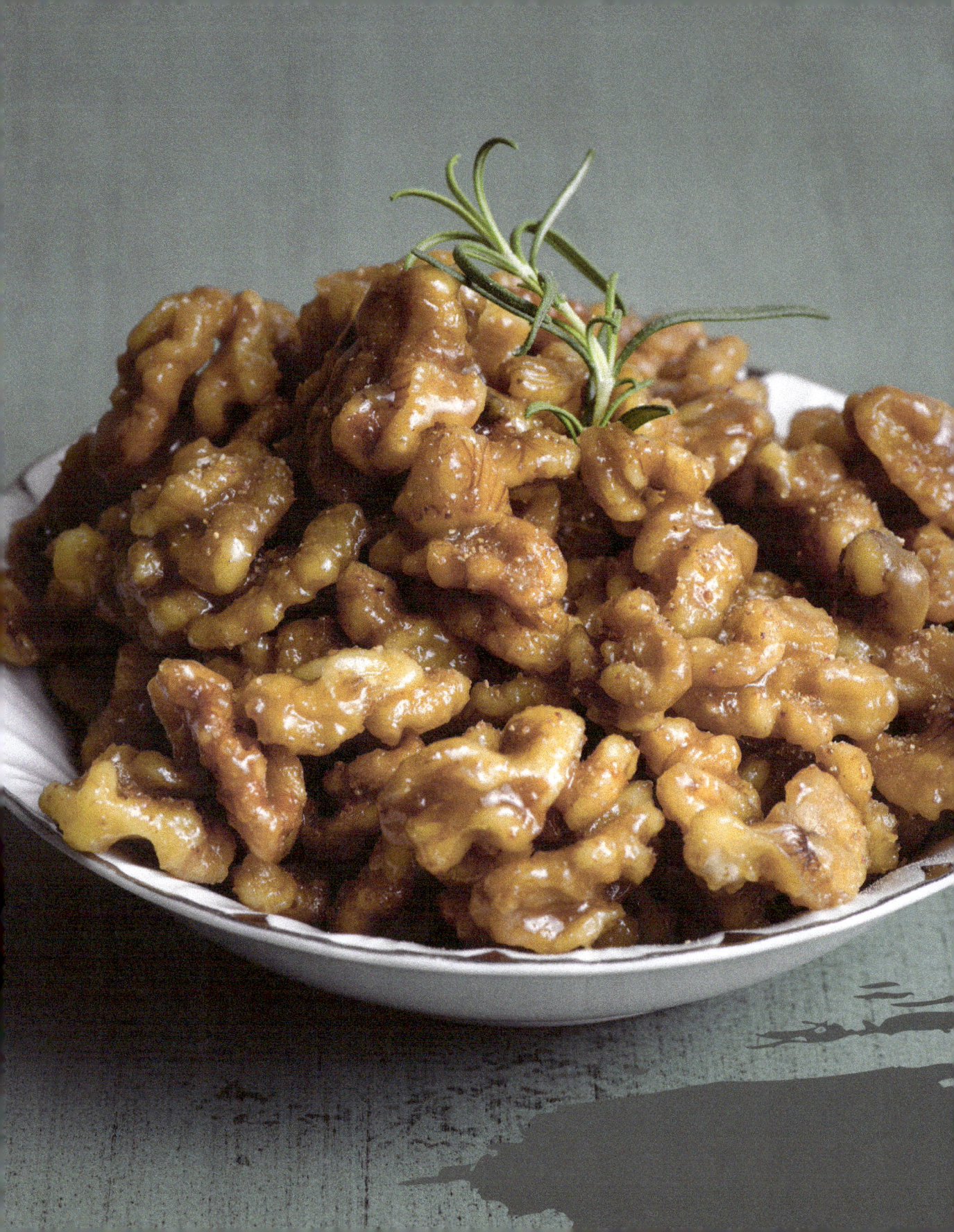

Candied Maple Walnuts

Kids' Favourite!

Serves 4

Ingredients:

- 2 cups walnuts, halved
- 1 Tbsp grapeseed or olive oil
- ½ cup organic maple syrup, or more to taste
- 1 tsp Celtic sea salt or Pink Himalayan salt
- 1 tsp maple or date sugar (optional)

Directions:

Preheat oven to 415 degrees. Rub first 3 ingredients together and put into a baking dish. Bake for 10-15 minutes until golden brown or even a tiny bit burnt looking. Remove from oven and sprinkle with salt and maple sugar (optional). Using a metal spatula, scrape the walnuts off the pan and combine gently with the melted maple syrup so that all of your pieces are well coated. Let cool. Scrape walnuts off again once cooled and place into a mason jar or other glass container and refrigerate immediately to keep the walnuts crisp and fresh. If you do not refrigerate them then they will be soft and sticky (not as delicous).

TRANSFORM

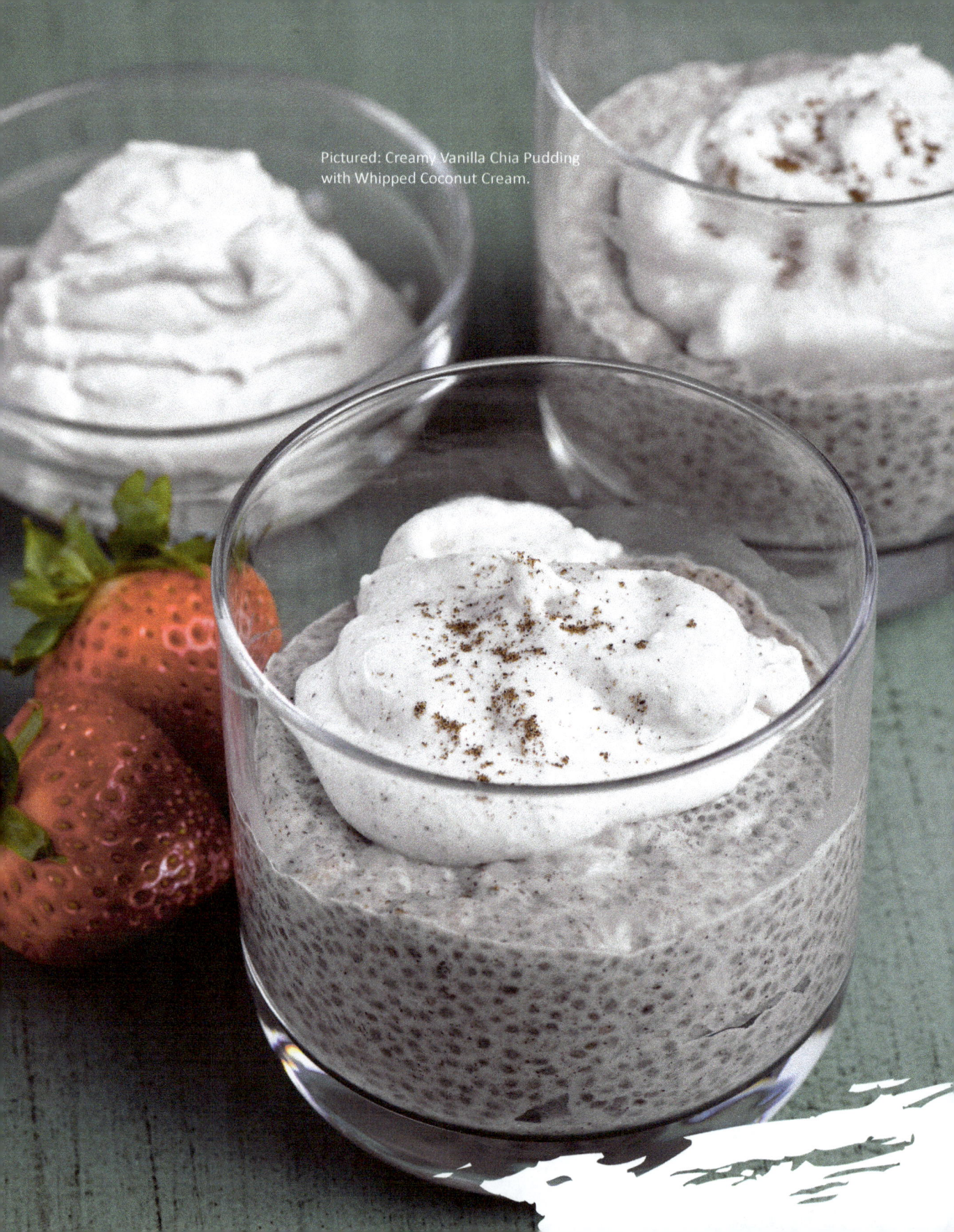

Pictured: Creamy Vanilla Chia Pudding with Whipped Coconut Cream.

Creamy Vanilla Chia Pudding

Kids' Favourite!

My little sister Ola introduced me to delicious and rich chia pudding and I've been experimenting with it ever since. This is a classic, rich, clean, vanilla pudding recipe to get you started, but feel free to try different variations. Makes 1 mason jar full, which is enough for 2 servings.

Serves 2

Ingredients:

- ½ cup full fat coconut milk from the can
- ½ cup unsweetened almond milk, flaxseed milk, cashew milk or other dairy milk alternative
- 3 Tbsp organic maple syrup or raw honey
- 1 tsp raw vanilla bean powder
- ¼ cup organic chia seeds
- A pinch of Celtic sea salt or Pink Himalayan salt

Directions:

Chia pudding needs time to set and thicken so make this recipe the night before and chill in the fridge overnight or for up to 3 days. The seeds will double in size and create a jelly-like outer surface. Combine all of the ingredients in a clear glass mason jar, with the chia seeds going in last, on top of everything else. Seal the jar and shake the ingredients together vigorously. If the chia isn't well blended, then open the jar and whisk the chia to combine. Place in the fridge to chill and thicken overnight. Serve with whipped coconut cream (recipe coming up) or top with fresh fruit, nuts or chocolate shavings.

Whipped Coconut Cream

Kids' Favourite!

This is a delicious non-dairy replacement for dairy whipped cream. Use it to garnish smoothies, baked bananas, fruit cups, or any other desert you love.

Ingredients:

- 1 can (14 oz) of full fat coconut milk
- 2 Tbsp organic maple syrup or raw honey
- 1 tsp raw vanilla bean powder

Directions:

Put the can of coconut milk in the fridge overnight (or for at least 10 hours). You want the cream (fat) to separate and solidify at the top. One hour before you are ready to make the whipped cream, put a metal bowl in your freezer to chill it. If you don't have a metal bowl, use a glass one (or use a larger glass Tupperware container). Take the can out of the fridge and flip it upside down. Open it up using a can opener and pour out the liquid so that there is nothing but the solid coconut cream left in the can. You can store the liquid from the top to use later in a smoothie if you want to. Scoop out the cream and place it into your chilled bowl. Using an electric hand mixer, beat the cream until it's smooth and fluffy. Then fold the maple syrup/honey and vanilla bean into it just to combine. Cover your bowl and put it back in the fridge until ready to serve. This recipe makes about 1 cup. It will last about 7 days in the fridge in a sealed container. Enjoy!!

Baked Cinnamon Apples

Kids' Favourite!

My Mom made this for us when we were children and I loved it very much then, and still do. This is a twist on the original, which used butter and white sugar. These are not chopped or sliced like most recipes, but left whole, and the cinnamon, coconut oil and maple sugar goodness erupts out from the centre as they bake.

Serves 4

Ingredients:

- 4 organic Macintosh or Spartan apples (conventional apples are heavily sprayed with pesticides so go organic)
- 2 Tbsp cinnamon
- 2 Tbsp maple sugar or coconut sugar
- 4 tsp virgin coconut oil
- A pinch of Celtic sea salt or Pink Himalayan salt

Directions:

Preheat your oven to 375 degrees. Wash your apples and pat dry. Using an apple corer, or anything else you have if you want to be creative, core the apples from the top, pulling out the seeds and tough core, but leaving the bottom of the apple in place. Basically, do not cut all the way through the centre of the apple to the other side, instead, leave about half a centimetre at the bottom to plug your hole. Place your apples on an oiled baking sheet, cored side up. In a cup or small bowl, combine the cinnamon, sugar, coconut oil and sea salt. Using a small spoon, spoon your cinnamon mixture into the hole so it's almost totally filled. Then take a teaspoon of coconut oil and pour it into the apple. Do that for all 4. Place the apples in the oven and bake for 30 minutes. The goodness in the centre will heat up and erupt gently over the top rim of the apple. Remove from oven and cool briefly before serving.

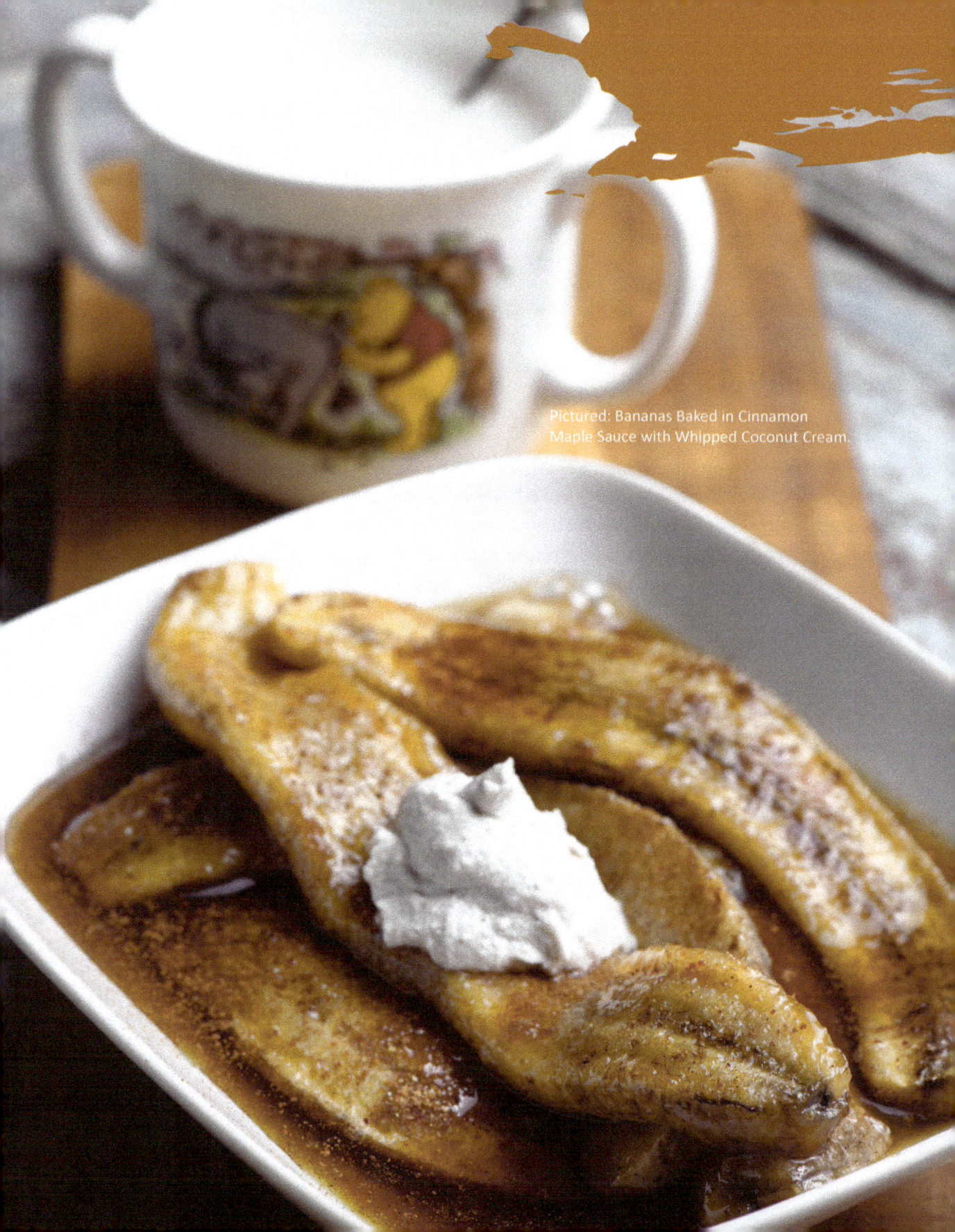

Pictured: Bananas Baked in Cinnamon Maple Sauce with Whipped Coconut Cream.

Bananas Baked in Cinnamon Maple Sauce

Kids' Favourite!

I absolutely love bananas. I discovered baked cinnamon bananas for breakfast in Cuba and it was like coming home to something I must have known my whole life. I don't know the recipe they used, but this is my version.

Serves 2

Ingredients:

- 4 ripe bananas
- ½ cup organic maple syrup
- 2 Tbsp maple or date sugar
- 1 Tbsp lemon juice
- 1 tsp cinnamon

Directions:

Preheat the oven to 375 degrees and get a non-stick baking pan out. Peel your bananas and cut them in half length-wise. Put them on your baking pan and rub them with maple syrup. Pour remaining maple syrup onto the top of the slices. Sprinkle with maple sugar, cinnamon and lemon juice. Pop into the oven and let bake for about 15 minutes. If you want to, you can bake them for 14 minutes and broil for 1. Serve hot with the maple sauce on top. Takes great with whipped coconut cream (see recipe on page 220) that has been blended with cinnamon.

Simple Fruit Salad with Omega Oil Sweet Sauce

Kids' Favourite!

This is a really great way to get omega oils into food that kids will love.

Serves 2

Ingredients:

- 2 cups of your favourite fruits, melons, berries
- ¼ cup Udo's Oil 3-6-9 Blend, hempseed oil or flaxseed oil
- ¼ cup organic maple syrup

Directions:

Mix all of the ingredients together and serve cold in small bowls. Stays fresh in the fridge for up to 3 days.

Warm Apple, Strawberry & Banana Crumble

Kids' Favourite!

Serves 4

Ingredients:

- Fruit filling:
- 2 large organic Macintosh Apples
- 2 cups of organic strawberries
- 1 banana
- 1 cup of pineapple juice or apple juice
- 1 Tbsp raw honey
- ½ tsp cinnamon
- A pinch of Celtic sea salt or Pink Himalayan salt

Crumble:
- 1 ½ cups rolled oats
- ½ cup of teff flour
- ¼ cup of organic maple syrup
- ¼ cup coconut oil, plus extra for oiling the baking dish
- ½ cup walnuts, chopped into small pieces
- ½ tsp cinnamon
- 1 tsp raw vanilla bean powder
- A pinch of Celtic sea salt or Pink Himalayan salt

Directions:

- Wash and dry apples. Peel the apples, cut out the cores and slice them up. Peel the banana and slice it up. Wash the strawberries, remove their tops, and slice into halves. Oil up a baking dish with coconut oil and place the fruit inside. Pour the pineapple juice over them and add a pinch of cinnamon and sea salt. Add honey and combine all ingredients together. To make the crumble, combine the oats, teff flour, maple syrup, coconut oil, walnuts, cinnamon, vanilla and pinch of sea salt in a bowl. Evenly distribute the crumble over the fruit mixture in the baking dish and bake for 30-40 minutes or until the topping is golden brown and crunchy and the fruit is soft and bubbling. Serve warm with a side of whipped coconut cream (see my recipe on page 220).

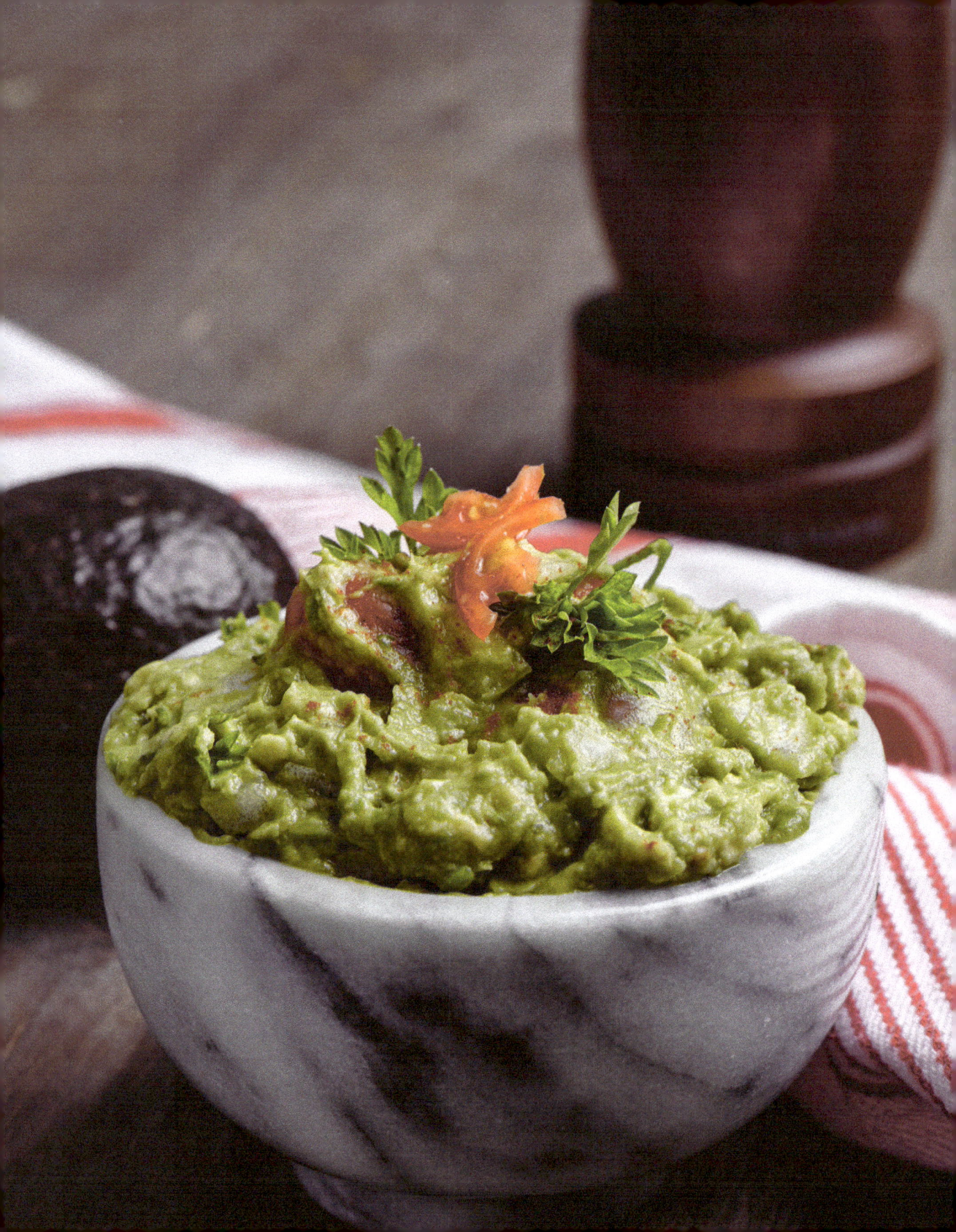

HOLY GUACAMOLE!

Kids' Favourite!

I know a young man who dreams of being a professional soccer player and, every time I see him, without fail, he asks me if I have some of my guacamole for him. This recipe is for you, Aidan.

Serves 2

INGREDIENTS:

- 2 avocados
- ¼ onion, finely chopped
- 7 Cherry tomatoes, chopped in half, or 1 small ripe Plum or Roma tomato, chopped into small pieces
- ¼ cup cilantro or parsley leaves, chopped
- Juice of 1 lime or lemon
- ½ tsp jalapeño pepper, seeded and chopped (optional)
- ½ tsp Celtic sea salt or Pink Himalayan salt
- ½ tsp smoked paprika
- ½ tsp cracked black pepper

DIRECTIONS:

Cut avocados in half, lengthwise, and use a spoon to scoop out the seed. Scoop out the flesh and put it into a bowl. Add lime juice and mash with a fork. Add all the rest of the ingredients and stir to combine. Serve immediately. Goes wonderfully on sprouted grain toast, on a sandwich, on top of mixed baby greens or tomatoes, as a veggie dip, as an ingredient in a salad dressing, with fish, or on its own as a salad or snack.

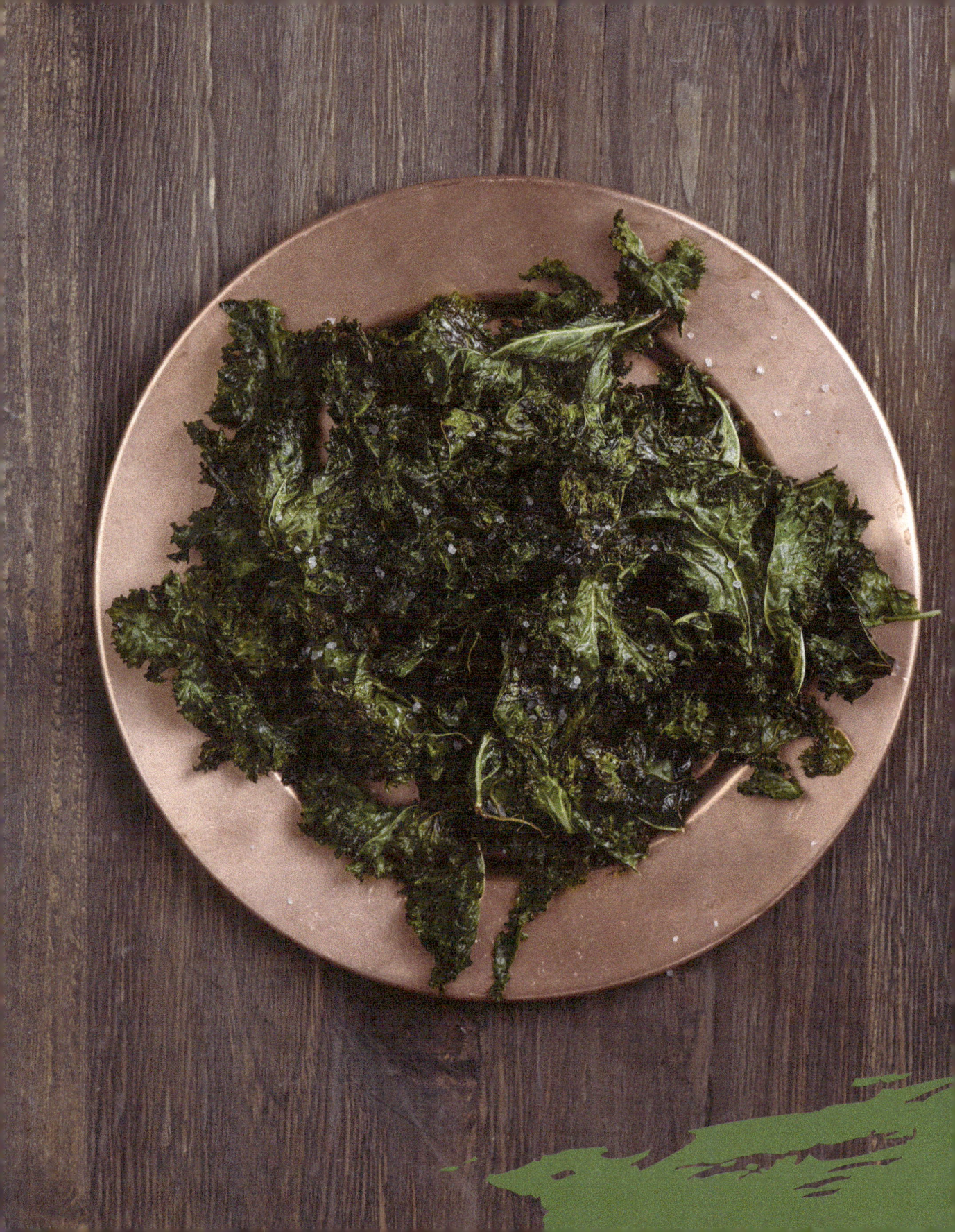

Kale Chips

Kids' Favourite!

If you don't know exactly what to do with the kale you bought, I would recommend trying this as your first kale recipe ever. It's genuinely healthy and genuinely tastes like junk food.

Serves 4

Ingredients:

- 1 bunch fresh kale
- 2 Tbsp olive oil for roasting or grapeseed oil
- ½ tsp Celtic sea salt or Pink Himalayan salt

Directions:

Preheat oven to 350 degrees. Wash kale and dry thoroughly. Remove the ribs from the kale and tear or cut the rest into pieces the size of your pinkie finger. Put onto a large baking dish and rub with oil and sprinkle with sea salt. Bake for about 15-20 minutes. Remove from oven and let cool. Taste and add extra salt if needed. Serve cold as a snack.

Optional:

- You can make a variety of flavours by adding spices before baking. Some suggestions would be garlic powder, Chili powder, cayenne pepper, smoked paprika, onion powder, steak spice, Cajun seasoning. Have fun with it!

Sweet Potato Fries

Kids' Favourite!

Serves 2

Ingredients:

- 2 large sweet potatoes
- 3 Tbsp extra virgin olive oil
- ½ tsp Celtic sea salt or Pink Himalayan salt
- A pinch of cayenne pepper

Directions:

Preheat oven to 425 degrees. Peel the sweet potatoes and cut into strips. Toss the sweet potatoes in the oil, salt and pepper. Spread them onto a baking dish, making sure they aren't piled on top of each other. Bake for 15 minutes and then take out of the oven and turn over. Bake for 10 more minutes, or until brown and crispy on the outside. Serve hot. Taste great with homemade mayonnaise made from Udo's Oil 3-6-9 Blend.

TRANSFORM 231

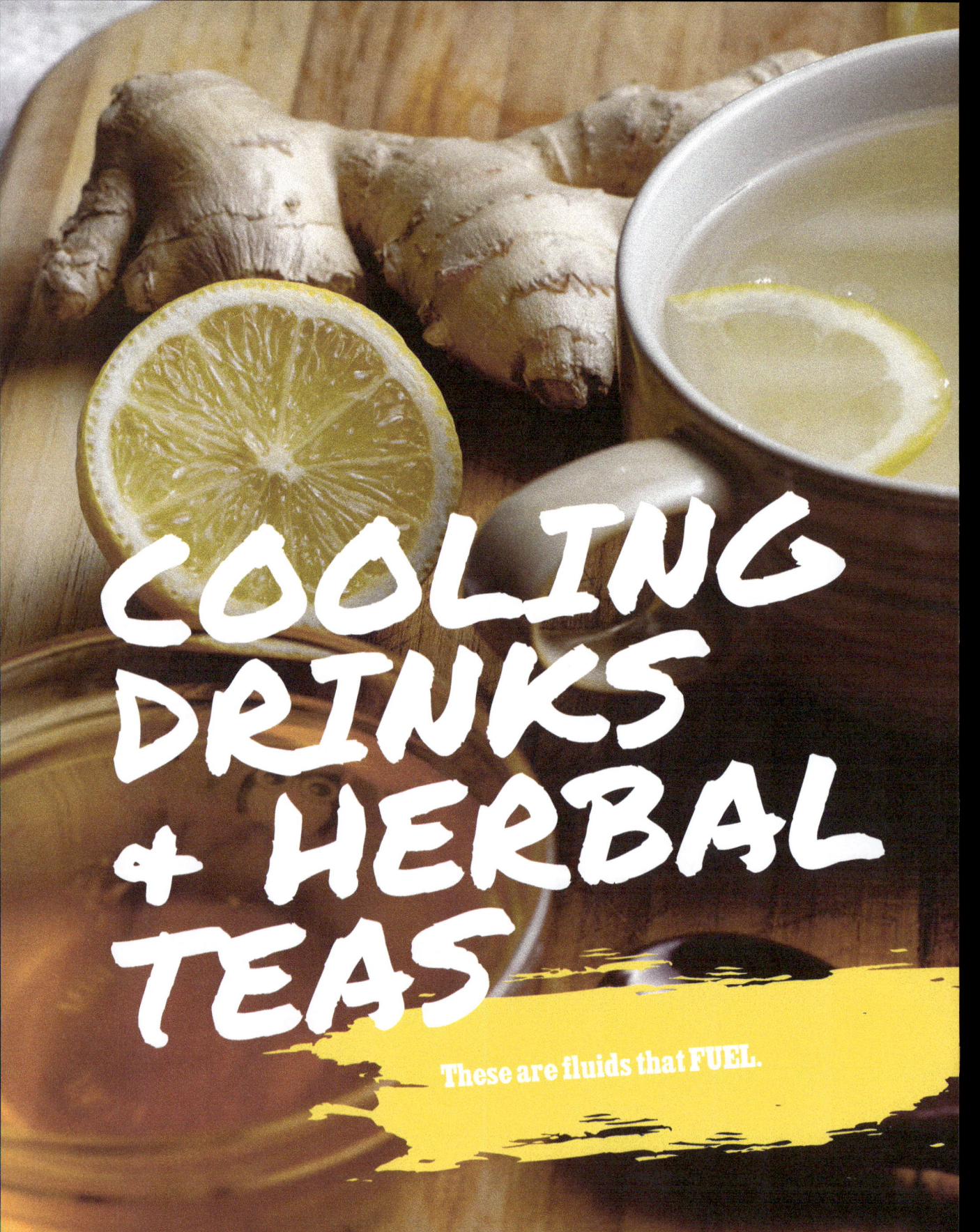

COOLING DRINKS & HERBAL TEAS

These are fluids that **FUEL**.

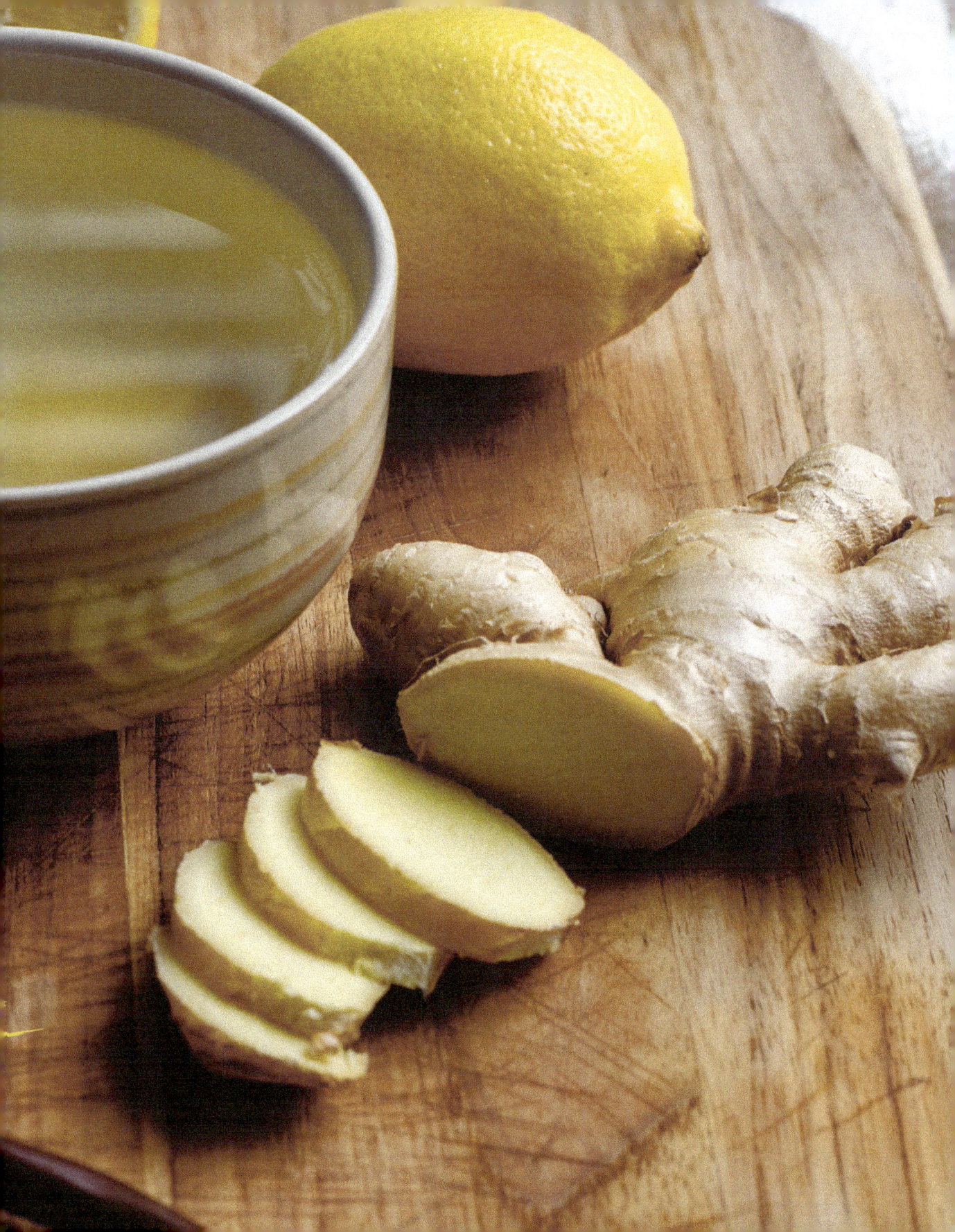

LEMONADE

Kids' Favourite!

Lemons have a cleansing and detoxifying effect on the body.

Serves 6

INGREDIENTS:

- 1 ½ cups freshly squeezed lemon juice
- 6 cups water
- 1 cup raw honey, more or less to sweeten

DIRECTIONS:

Combine all ingredients together in a jug and serve chilled.

Spinach, Green Apple & Ginger Revitalizer

This is a great pick-me-up, packed with energy.

Serves 1

Ingredients:

- 1 cup baby spinach leaves
- ¾ green apple, chopped
- 1 inch piece of ginger root, peeled and chopped into pieces
- 1 cup pineapple juice
- ½ cup water

Directions:

To make, combine all ingredients in a blender and blend until well combined. Blend in a bit of ice if you'd like it to be colder. Serve immediately in a mason jar. Swish around in your mouth before swallowing.

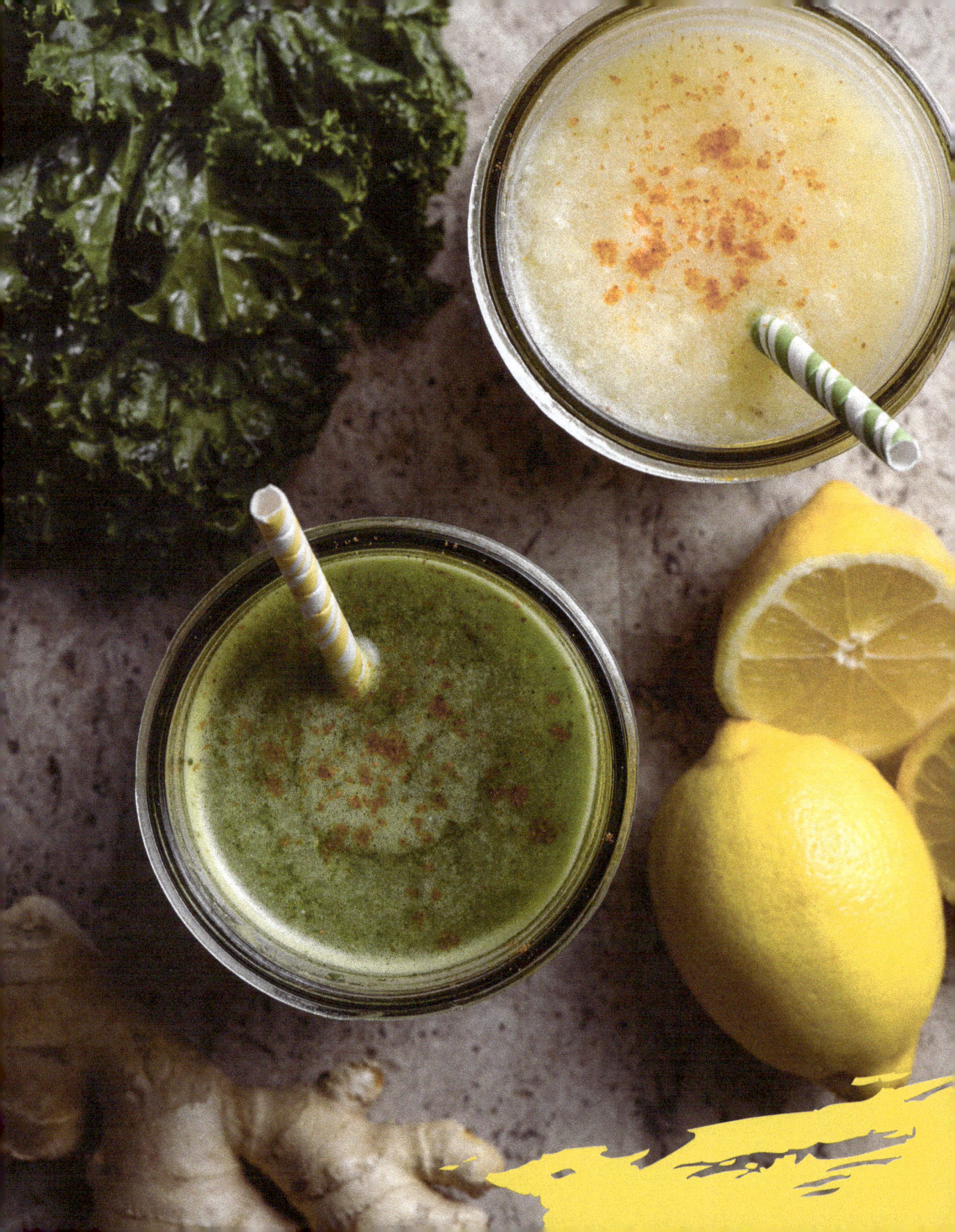

CAYENNE KICKER

This has some serious *POW* and is not for the meek! Take this in the morning to cleanse the body as a shot (reduce the amount of liquid significantly and halve the ingredients) or as a drink (make as instructed below). If taking as a drink, swish around in your mouth before swallowing every time. Below are 3 of my favourite varieties. To make, combine all ingredients in a blender, including the whole chunks of lemon (do not juice it) and blend until well combined. Blend in a bit of ice if you'd like it to be colder. Serve immediately in a mason jar or shot glass.

Serves 1

INGREDIENTS:

Original Kicker:

- 2 lemons, peeled and cut in half
- 1 inch piece of ginger root, peeled and chopped into pieces
- 1 Tbsp raw honey
- A dash of organic cayenne pepper
- 1 ¼ cup water

Pineapple Grapefruit Kicker:

- 2 lemons, peeled and cut in half
- 1 inch piece of ginger root, peeled and chopped into pieces
- ½ grapefruit, cut into chunks
- ½ cup pineapple chunks
- 1 Tbsp raw honey
- A dash of organic cayenne pepper
- 1 ¼ cup water

Kale Kicker:

- 2 lemons, peeled and cut in half
- 1 inch piece of ginger root, peeled and chopped into pieces
- ½ cup kale
- ½ cup pineapple chunks
- 1 Tbsp raw honey
- A dash of organic cayenne pepper
- 1 ¼ cup water

Get Well Drink

The name says it all.

Serves 1

Ingredients:

- 2 small carrots or 1 big one, peeled
- ½ green apple, chopped
- ½ cup baby spinach leaves
- ½ cup pineapple chunks
- 1 cup pineapple juice
- ½ cup water

Directions:

To make, combine all ingredients in a blender and blend until well combined. Blend in a bit of ice if you'd like it to be colder. Serve immediately in a mason jar. Swish around in your mouth before swallowing.

The Healthy Start

This was a mistake I made that ended up being a hit. It's loaded with powerful foods too.

Serves 2

Ingredients:

- ½ cup mango chunks
- 1 inch piece of ginger root, peeled and chopped into pieces
- ½ cup pineapple chunks
- ½ grapefruit, cut into chunks
- ½ cup parsley, chopped
- 1 ½ cups water
- 1 Tbsp raw honey, or more to taste

Directions:

To make, combine all ingredients in a blender and blend until well combined. Blend in a bit of ice if you'd like it to be colder. Serve immediately in a mason jar. Swish around in your mouth before swallowing.

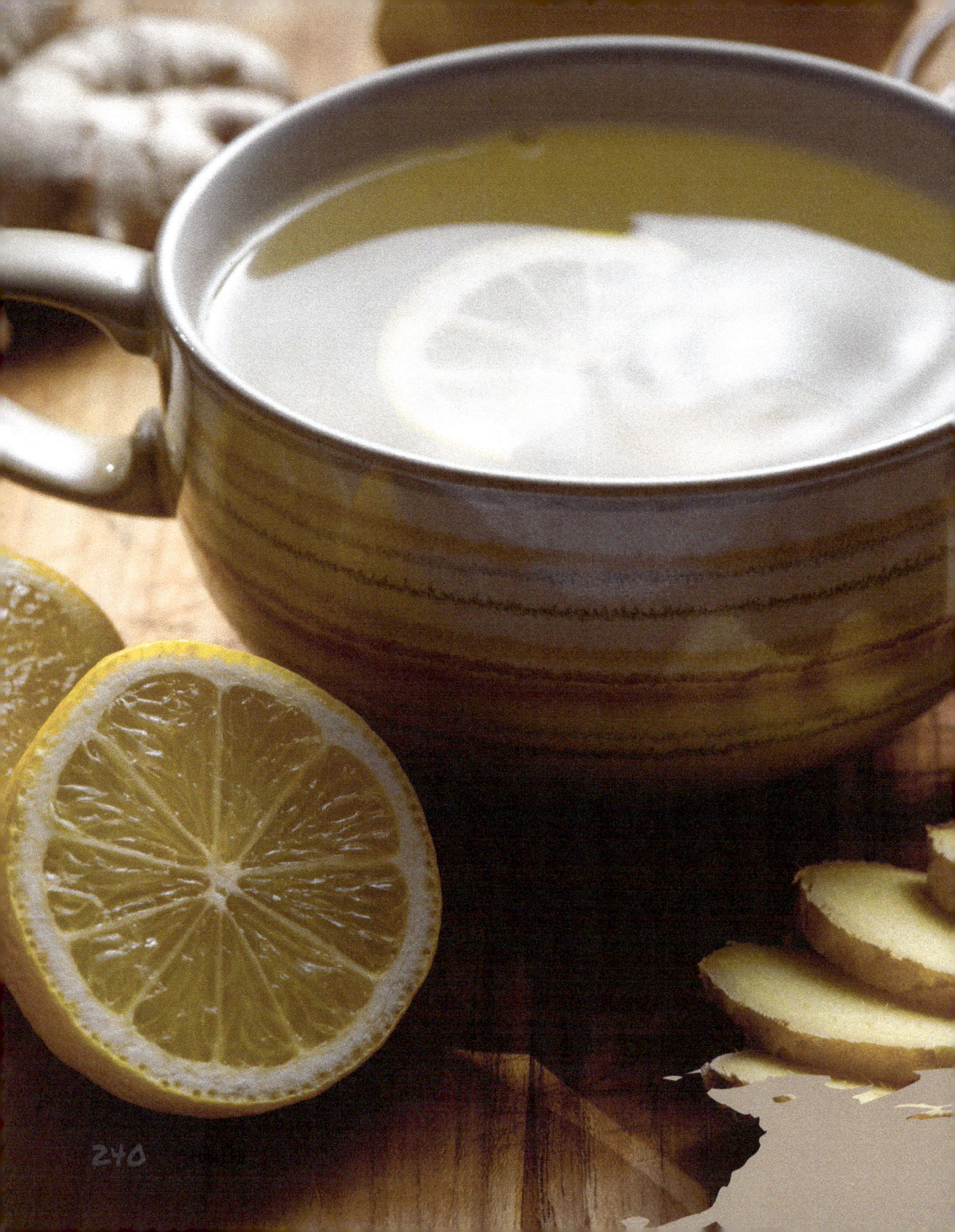

Ginger Tea

Kids' Favourite!

This helps your stomach feel better, helps you digest food, boosts your immune system and fights colds. Don't buy the packaged one, the homemade version is so easy. Ginger is an herb, not a tea leaf, and does not contain any caffeine.

Serves 2

Ingredients:

- Piece of ginger root the size of your pinkie finger, peeled and chopped into pieces
- 1 ½ - 2 cups water
- Juice of ½ lemon (optional)
- 1 Tbsp raw honey, or to taste

Directions:

Put ginger and water together in a saucepan. Boil for 20 minutes on medium heat. Add lemon and honey just before serving. Serve hot. Store leftovers in the fridge for up to 2 days.

Mint Tea with Honey

Mint is a very cleansing herb, it helps indigestion and cleanses your breath. It is also very high in antioxidants. Mint is an herb, not a tea leaf, and does not contain any caffeine.

Serves 1

Ingredients:

- 10 mint leaves
- 1 ½ - 2 cups water
- 1 Tbsp raw honey, or to taste

Directions:

Boil mint and water together in a saucepan for 10 minutes. Remove from heat and add honey to it just before serving. Store leftovers in the fridge for up to 2 days.

Hibiscus & Mint Tea with Frozen Pineapple & Honey

Hibiscus tea has an incredible dark red colour and has traditionally been used to improve blood circulation and cardiovascular health. Coupled with mint, this packs a powerful health punch. Both hibiscus and mint are not real tea leaves, they do not come from tea plants, and therefore are caffeine free "teas."

Serves 2

Ingredients:

- 1 Tbsp hibiscus or sorrel dried tea
- 5 mint leaves, or more to taste
- 5 chunks of frozen pineapple
- 2 cups water
- 1 Tbsp raw honey, or to taste

Directions:

Boil 2 cups of water on the stove. In a teapot, combine all of the other ingredients, except honey. Add boiled water. Steep for 5 minutes, but you can keep all the ingredients in the hot water indefinitely. Add honey and serve warm.

A Final Note

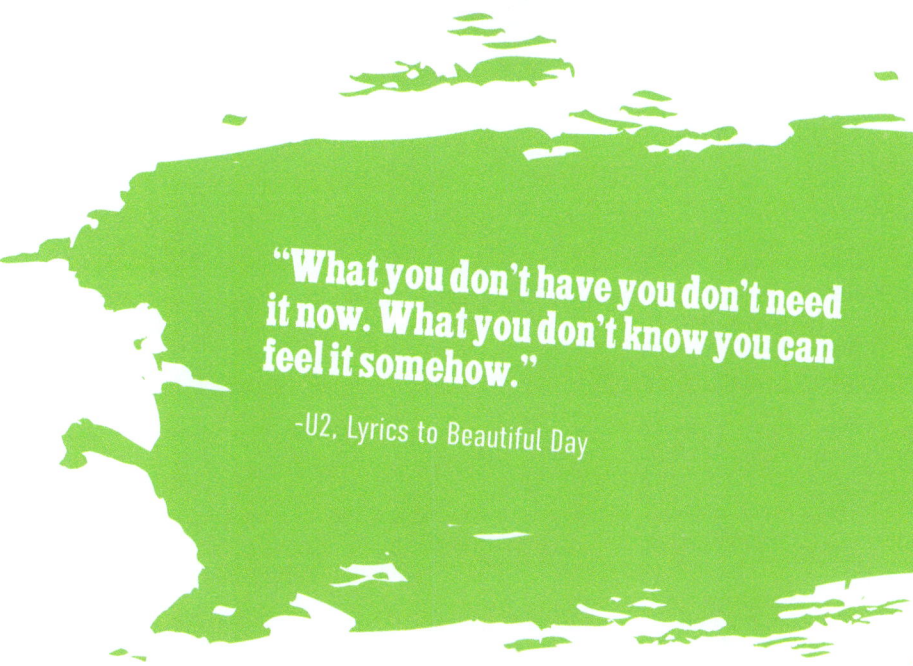

> "What you don't have you don't need it now. What you don't know you can feel it somehow."
>
> —U2, Lyrics to Beautiful Day

This is the end of the book. You now know what you need to know. There may be some more facts you'd like to learn about, but the fundamentals have been presented to you in this book. This is knowledge that has now become a part of you. That can never be taken away. Once you learn a new and revolutionary idea that transforms the way you view the world, it is yours forever. The fundamentals presented in the pages of this book, in *FUELLED*, are going to be there for you. You might wish to revisit them on a regular basis to remind yourself of what you have learned. And practice these principles, make these recipes, so that your mindset doesn't get rusty or your vision faded. And that way, once you start to walk the walk, I truly believe that life will show you the pieces that are still missing for you to create the life you want for yourself.

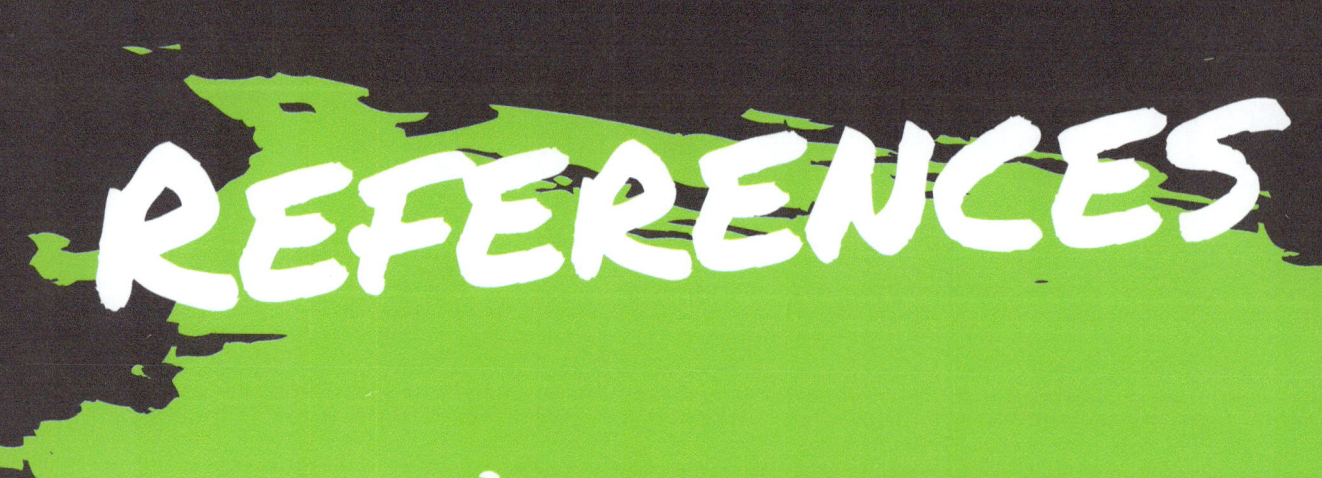

Stand on the shoulders of giants.

INTRODUCTION

Cvijetic, Z. (2016, December 26). 13 Things You Should Give Up If You Want To Be Successful. *Personal Growth, Medium*. Retrieved from http://medium.com/personal-growth/13-things-you-need-to-give-up-if-you-want-to-be-successful-44b5b9b06a26.

PART 1: EDUCATE
INTRO

Phoenix, J. (2017, March 14). Knowledge Is Power. *Uncommon Sense*. Retrieved from http://uncommonsense.is/post/19861932097/knowledge-is-power.

THE POWER OF THE HUMAN BODY/CELLS

A Super Brief and Basic Explanation of Epigenetics for Total Beginners. (2017, October 17). *What Is Epigenetics?*. Retrieved from www.whatisepigenetics.com/what-is-epigenetics/.

Babraham Institute. (2016, October 12). Vitamins A and C help erase cell memory: Discovery important in development of cells for regenerative medicine. *ScienceDaily*. Retrieved from www.sciencedaily.com/releases/2016/10/161012132810.htm.

Boyanapalli, S. S. S., and Ah-Ng, T.K. (2015). Curcumin, the King of Spices': Epigenetic Regulatory Mechanisms in the Prevention of Cancer, Neurological, and Inflammatory Diseases. *Current Pharmacology Reports, 1(2)*, pp. 129–139. doi: 10.1007/s40495-015-0018-x or https://link.springer.com/content/pdf/10.1007%2Fs40495-015-0018-x.pdf

Burdge, G. C., et al. (2012). Epigenetics: Are There Implications for Personalised Nutrition? *Current Opinion in Clinical Nutrition and Metabolic Care, 15(5)*, pp. 442–447. doi: 10.1097/mco.0b013e3283567dd2.

Carey, N. (2012). *The Epigenetics Revolution: How Modern Biology Is Rewriting Our Understanding of Genetics, Disease, and Inheritance*. New York: Columbia University Press.

Choi, S.W, and Friso, S. (2010, November 1). Epigenetics: A New Bridge between Nutrition and Health. *Advances in Nutrition: An International Review Journal, 1*, pp. 8-16. Retrieved from doi: 10.3945/an.110.1004 or http://advances.nutrition.org/content/1/1/8.full.

Chopra, D. and Tanzi, R.E. (2015). *Super Genes: Unlock the Astonishing Power of Your DNA for Optimum Health and Well-Being*. New York: Harmony Books.

Dolinoy, D. C., et al. (2006).Maternal Genistein Alters Coat Color and Protects Avy Mouse Offspring from Obesity by Modifying the Fetal Epigenome. *Environmental Health Perspectives, 114 (4)*, pp. 567–572. Retrieved from doi: 10.1289/ehp.8700.

Epigenetics vs. Genetics. (2011, June 25). *Wassup, Doc?* Retrieved from: https://wassupdoc.wordpress.com/2011/06/25/epigenetics-vs-genetics/.

Hore, T. A., et al. (2016, November).Retinol and Ascorbate Drive Erasure of Epigenetic Memory and Enhance Reprogramming to Naive Pluripotency by Complementary Mechanisms. *Proceedings of the National Academy of Sciences, 113(43)*, pp. 12202–12207. Retrieved from doi: 10.1073/pnas.1608679113.

Jaenisch, R. and Bird, A. (2003, March 1). Epigenetic Regulation of Gene Expression: How the Genome Integrates Intrinsic and Environmental Signals. *Nature Genetics, 33*, pp. 245–254. Retrieved from doi: 10.1038/ng1089.

Kucharski, R., et al. (2008, March 28). Nutritional Control of Reproductive Status in Honeybees via DNA Methylation. *Science, 319(5871),* pp. 1827–1830. Retrieved from doi: 10.1126/science.1153069.

Lumey, L., et al. (2007). Cohort Profile: The Dutch Hunger Winter Families Study. *International Journal of Epidemiology, 36(6),* pp. 1196–1204. Retrieved from doi: 10.1093/ije/dym126.

Mercola, Joseph. (2016). *Effortless Healing: 9 Simple Ways to Sidestep Illness, Shed Excess Weight, and Help Your Body Fix Itself.* New York: Harmony Crown.

Reuter, S., et al. (2011). Epigenetic Changes Induced by Curcumin and Other Natural Compounds. *Genes & Nutrition, 6(2),* pp. 93–108. Retrieved from doi: 10.1007/s12263-011-0222-1.

Rijlaarsdam, J., et al. (2016). Prenatal Unhealthy Diet, Insulin-like Growth Factor 2 Gene (IGF2) Methylation, and Attention Deficit Hyperactivity Disorder Symptoms in Youth with Early-Onset Conduct Problems. *Journal of Child Psychology and Psychiatry, 58(1),* pp. 19–27. Retrieved from doi:10.1111/jcpp.12589.

Sinclair, K. D., et al. (2007, October). DNA Methylation, Insulin Resistance, and Blood Pressure in Offspring Determined by Maternal Periconceptional B Vitamin and Methionine Status. *PNAS, 104(49),* pp. 19351–19356. Retrieved from doi: 10.1073/pnas.0707258104.

Wargovich, M. J. (1997). Experimental Evidence for Cancer Preventive Elements in Foods. *Cancer Letters, 114(1-2),* pp. 11–17. Retrieved from doi: 10.1016/s0304-3835(97)04616-8.

Weaver, I. C., et al. (2004, June 27). Epigenetic Programming by Maternal Behavior. *Nature Neuroscience, 7,* pp. 847–854. Retrieved from doi: 10.1038/nn1276.

Wilken, R., et al. (2011). Curcumin: A Review of Anti-Cancer Properties and Therapeutic Activity in Head and Neck Squamous Cell Carcinoma. *Molecular Cancer, 10(1),* p. 12. Retrieved from doi: 10.1186/1476-4598-10-12.

Zhong, J., et al. (2017, April 18). B Vitamins Attenuate the Epigenetic Effects of Ambient Fine Particles in a Pilot Human Intervention Trial. *PNAS, 114(16),* pp. 3505–3508. Retrieved from doi: 10.1073/pnas.1618545114.

MASTERING OUR BODY COMES FIRST

Chopra, D. and Tanzi, R.E. (2015). *Super Genes: Unlock the Astonishing Power of Your DNA for Optimum Health and Well-Being.* New York: Harmony Books.

Maslow, A. H. (1943). A Theory of Human Motivation. *Psychological Review, 50(4),* pp. 370-396.

Maslow, A. H. (1954). *Motivation and Personality.* New York: Harper & Row.

Tie It All Together. (2017, August 30). *Tonyrobbins.com.* Retrieved from www.tonyrobbins.com/leadership-impact/tie-it-all-together/.

YOUR PHILOSOPHY ON HEALTH, ENERGY AND EATING

Robbins, T. (2016). *Life Mastery Workbook.* Fiji.

WHAT THE BODY NEEDS TO STAY HEALTHY

Link, R. (2017, September 15). 11 Essential Nutrients Your Body Needs Now. *Dr. Axe.* Retrieved from draxe.com/essential-nutrients/.

Robbins, T. (2016). Vital Components of Health. *Life Mastery Workbook.* Fiji.

Sizer, F.S., Whitney, E., and Piche, L.A. (2012). *Nutrition: Concepts and Controversies* (2nd Canadian edition). Toronto: Nelson Education.

WONDERS OF WATER

Batmanghelidj, F. (2003). *Water: for Health, for Healing, for Life: You're Not Sick, You're Thirsty!.* New York: Warner Books.

Batmanghelidj, F. (2008). You're Not Sick; You're Thirsty. Don't Treat Thirst with Medication. *WaterCure | The Miracles of Water to Cure Diseases.* Retrieved from www.watercure.com/.

Mercola, J. (2016). *Effortless Healing: 9 Simple Ways to Sidestep Illness, Shed Excess Weight, and Help Your Body Fix Itself.* New York: Harmony Crown.

FOCUSING ON YOUR FOUNDATION

Environmental Working Group (2017). *EWG*. Retrieved from www.ewg.org/.

Health Canada. (2008, January 14).Vegetables and Fruit. *Canada.ca*. Retrieved from www.canada.ca/en/health-canada/services/food-nutrition/canada-food-guide/choosing-foods/vegetables-fruit.html.

Mercola, J. (2016). *Effortless Healing: 9 Simple Ways to Sidestep Illness, Shed Excess Weight, and Help Your Body Fix Itself*. New York: Harmony Crown.

PLU Code News (2014-2015).*PLU-Codes*. Retrieved from www.ifpsglobal.com/Identification/PLU-Codes.

PLU Database. (2014-2015). *PLU-Codes Search*, International Federation for Produce Standards,, Retrieved from www.ifpsglobal.com/Identification/PLU-Codes/PLU-codes-Search.

Produce IFPS PLU Codes: A User's Guide. (2016, September). *IFPS Global*, International Federation for Produce Standards. Retrieved from www.ifpsglobal.com/Portals/22/IFPS%20Documents/PLU%20User%20guides/PLU%20Users%20Guide%20Sept%202016.pdf?ver=2016-09-23-144820-713.

Wolfe, D. (2009). *Superfoods: The food and medicine of the future*. Berkeley, California: North Atlantic Books.

HEALTHY (AND DOWN RIGHT ESSENTIAL) FATS AND OILS

Erasmus, U. (2012). Dr. Udo Erasmus on Living Healthier: The father of omega-3 and healthy fats and author of Fats That Heal, Fats That Kill, Diet and Fitness Expert, *First30Days*. Retrieved from www.first30days.com/experts/dr-udo-erasmus.

Erasmus, U. (1993). *Fats that heal, fats that kill: The complete guide to fats, oils, cholesterol and human health*. Burnaby: Alive Books Publishing.

Hyman, M. (2017). Eat Fat, Get Thin: The Surprising Truth About the Fat We Eat - the Key to Sustained Weight Loss and Vibrant Health. Retrieved from drhyman.com/wp-content/uploads/2015/04/EFGT-Manual-PDF.

Munoz, K. (2017, August 9). The 5 Best Healthy Fats for Your Body. *Dr. Axe*. Retrieved from draxe.com/healthy-fats/.

Sacks, F. M., et al. (2017, January 1). Dietary Fats and Cardiovascular Disease: A Presidential Advisory From the American Heart Association. *Circulation, American Heart Association, Inc*. Retrieved from circ.ahajournals.org/content/early/2017/06/15/CIR.0000000000000510.

United States Federal Government. (1980). Nutrition and Your Health: Dietary Guidelines for Americans. Retrieved from health.gov/dietaryguidelines/1980.asp.

PERFECT PROTEINS

Health Canada. (2017, February 3). Mercury in Fish. *Canada.ca*. Retrieved from www.canada.ca/en/health-canada/services/food-nutrition/food-safety/chemical-contaminants/environmental-contaminants/mercury/mercury-fish.html.

Health Canada. (2012, November 19). Meat and Alternatives. *Canada.ca*. www.canada.ca/en/health-canada/services/food-nutrition/canada-food-guide/choosing-foods/meat-alternatives.html.

Health Canada. (2016, September 1). Canada's Food Guides. *Canada.ca*. Retrieved from www.canada.ca/en/health-canada/services/canada-food-guides.html.

Consumers. (2017). Consumer Resources to Support Sustainable Seafood from the Seafood Watch Program at the Monterey Bay Aquarium. Retrieved from www.seafoodwatch.org/consumers.

Consumer Guides. (2017). Printable Consumer Guides with Seafood and Sushi Recommendations from the Seafood Watch Program at the Monterey Bay Aquarium. Retrieved from www.seafoodwatch.org/seafood-recommendations/consumer-guides.

Erasmus, U. (1993). *Fats that heal, fats that kill: The complete guide to fats, oils, cholesterol and human health*. Burnaby: Alive Books Publishing.

Exceptional Care for Exceptional Animals. (2017). *Monterey Bay Aquarium – Official Site*, www.montereybayaquarium.org/.

Munoz, K. (2017, August 9). The 5 Best Healthy Fats for Your Body. *Dr. Axe*. Retrieved from draxe.com/healthy-fats/.

Mercola, J. (2017). *Fat for Fuel: a Revolutionary Diet to Combat Cancer, Boost Brain Power, and Increase Your Energy*. USA: Hay House.

Science Study Predicts Collapse of All Seafood Fisheries by 2050.(2006, November 2). *Stanford University*. Retrieved from news.stanford.edu/news/2006/november8/ocean-110806.html.

Sizer, F.S., Whitney, E., and Piche, L.A. (2012). *Nutrition: Concepts and Controversies* (2nd Canadian edition). Toronto: Nelson Education.

USDA. (2016, October 3). Americans' Seafood Consumption Below Recommendations. *USDA ERS* - Retrieved from www.ers.usda.gov/amber-waves/2016/october/americans-seafood-consumption-below-recommendations/.

USDA. (2017a). Food Availability (Per Capita) Data System. *USDA ERS - Food Availability (Per Capita) Data System*. Retrieved from www.ers.usda.gov/data-products/food-availability-per-capita-data-system/

USDA. (2017b). Nutrient Content and Variability in Newly Obtained Salmon Data for USDA Nutrient Database for Standard Reference. Retrieved from www.ars.usda.gov/ARSUserFiles/80400525/Articles/EB07_Salmon.pdf.

USDA. (2017c). Sunflower Seed Butter and Almond Butter as Nutrient-Rich Alternatives to Peanut Butter. Retrieved from www.ars.usda.gov/ARSUserFiles/80400525/Articles/ADA10_SunflowerAlmondButter.pdf.

USDA. (2017d). USDA Foods Product Information Sheet: 110854 - Peanut Butter, Individual Portion. Retrieved from fns-prod.azureedge.net/sites/default/files/fdd/110854-peanut-butter.pdf.

HERBS, FERMENTED FOODS & BETTER SWEETENERS

Mercola, J. (2016). *Effortless Healing: 9 Simple Ways to Sidestep Illness, Shed Excess Weight, and Help Your Body Fix Itself*. New York: Harmony Crown.

Wolfe, D. (2009). *Superfoods: The food and medicine of the future*. Berkeley, California: North Atlantic Books.

ON EATING MEAT

Government of Canada, Canadian Food Inspection Agency, Food Labelling and Claims Directorate. (2016, January 12). Information within the Nutrition Facts Table. Retrieved from www.inspection.gc.ca/food/labelling/food-labelling-for-industry/nutrition-labelling/information-within-the-nutrition-facts-table/eng/1389198568400/1389198597278?chap=6.

Health Canada. (2012, November 19). Meat and Alternatives. *Canada.ca*. Retrieved from www.canada.ca/en/health-canada/services/food-nutrition/canada-food-guide/choosing-foods/meat-alternatives.html.

Scientific Report of the 2015 Dietary Guidelines Advisory Committee. (2015). *ASDA*. Retrieved from health.gov/dietaryguidelines/2015-scientific-report/pdfs/scientific-report-of-the-2015-dietary-guidelines-advisory-committee.pdf.

SUPPLEMENTS

Axe, J. (2017, June 21). Is Your Multi-Vitamin Helping or Hurting You?" *Dr. Axe*. Retrieved from draxe.com/is-your-multi-vitamin-helping-or-hurting-you/.

Boldt, E. (2017, October 6). Absorb More Nutrients with Digestive Enzymes. *Dr. Axe*. Retreived from draxe.com/digestive-enzymes/.

Chopra, D. and Tanzi, R.E. (2015). *Super Genes: Unlock the Astonishing Power of Your DNA for Optimum Health and Well-Being*. New York: Harmony Books.

Dietary Supplements - Safe, Beneficial and Regulated. (2017, July). *Council for Responsible Nutrition*, Retrieved from www.crnusa.org/resources/dietary-supplements-safe-beneficial-and-regulated.

Dietary Supplements: What You Need to Know. (2011). *NIH Office of Dietary Supplements, U.S. Department of Health and Human Services*. Retrieved from ods.od.nih.gov/HealthInformation/DS_WhatYouNeedToKnow.aspx.

Dietary Supplement Fact Sheets. *NIH Office of Dietary Supplements, U.S. Department of Health and Human Services*. Retrieved from ods.od.nih.gov/factsheets/list-all/.

Government of Canada, Canadian Food Inspection Agency, Food Labelling and Claims Directorate. (2016, January 12). Information within the Nutrition Facts Table. Retrieved from www.inspection.gc.ca/food/labelling/food-labelling-for-industry/nutrition-labelling/information-within-the-nutrition-facts-table/eng/1389198568400/1389198597278?chap=6.

Government of Canada, Health Canada, Health Products and Food Branch, Natural Health Products Directorate. (2016, December 8).Common Menu Bar Links. *Questions from Consumers - Regulation of Natural Health Products*. Retrieved from www.hc-sc.gc.ca/dhp-mps/prodnatur/faq/question_consum-consom-eng.php.

Health Canada. (2015, February 25). Nutrients in Food. *Canada.ca*. Retrieved from www.canada.ca/en/health-canada/services/nutrients.html.

Mercola, J. (2016). *Effortless Healing: 9 Simple Ways to Sidestep Illness, Shed Excess Weight, and Help Your Body Fix Itself*. New York: Harmony Crown.

Pudell, C., et al. (2013, November 6). Fish Oil Improves Anxiety-like, Depressive-like and Cognitive Behaviors in Olfactory Bulbectomised Rats. *European Journal of Neuroscience*, 39(2), pp. 266–274. Retrieved from doi: 10.1111/ejn.12406.

Weeks, C. (2016, September 9). Health Canada to Change Standards for Natural Health Products. *The Globe and Mail*. Retrieved from https://beta.theglobeandmail.com/news/national/health-canada-to-change-standards-for-natural-health-products/article31810843/?ref=http%3A%2F%2Fwww.theglobeandmail.com&.

IT MIGHT SEEM HARD BUT...

Kondo, M. (2014). *The Life-Changing Magic of Tidying up: the Japanese Art of Decluttering and Organizing* (1st ed.). Berkeley: Ten Speed Press.

ELIMINATION DIETS

Health Canada. (2012, August 22). Food Allergies and Intolerances. *Canada.ca*. Retrieved from www.canada.ca/en/health-canada/services/food-nutrition/food-safety/food-allergies-intolerances.html.

Health Canada. (2009, June 9). Food Allergies. *Canada.ca*. Retrieved from https://www.canada.ca/en/health-canada/services/healthy-living/your-health/food-nutrition/food-allergies.html.

Hyman, M. (2017, May 8). 10 Steps to Reverse Autoimmune Disease. Retrieved from www.drhyman.com/blog/2015/09/04/10-steps-to-reverse-autoimmune-disease/.

Walsh, B. (2016, May 9). Food Sensitivities and Intolerances: How and Why to Do an Elimination Diet. *Precision Nutrition*. Retrieved from www.precisionnutrition.com/elimination-diet.

90/10 RULE FOR SUCCESS

Rosenthal, J. M. (2008). *Integrative Nutrition: Feed Your Hunger for Health and Happiness*. New York: Integrative Nutrition Publishing.

Hunter, J.J. (2017). What Is The 90/10 Rule? 9010 LIFE Explained. Retrieved from http://jeffjhunter.com/9010-rule-9010-life/.

DELICIOUS!

Adler, T. (2015, October 11). Are Vegetables the New Meat? One Writer Assesses the Chef-Driven, Plant-Centric Gastronomic Boom. *Vogue*. Retrieved from www.vogue.com/article/are-vegetables-the-new-meat.

LIFESTYLE RECOMMENDATIONS

Hendricks, G. (2011). *Learning to Love Yourself*. USA: Createspace Independent Publishing Platform.

Peets Jr., E. (2015). *Sunday to Sunday 40-Day Devotional: Healing for Old Wounds. Grace for the Journey*. USA: Xulon Press.

PART 2: INSPIRE
INTRODUCTION

Hill, N. (2007). *Think and Grow Rich: Original 1937 Classic Edition*. USA: Marketplace Books.

Osteen, J. (2012, October 28). Pastor Joel Osteen's Full Sermon "The Power of 'I Am.'" *Oprah Winfrey Network*. Retrieved from www.youtube.com/watch?v=_kjSK-PcU9o.

Phoenix, J. (2016, February 25). Fuck Your Comfort Zone. *Uncommon Sense*. Retrieved from uncommonsense.is/post/69926233954/fuck-your-comfort-zone.

OVERCOMING FEAR

Cvijetic, Z. (2016, December 26). 13 Things You Should Give Up If You Want To Be Successful. *Personal Growth, Medium*. Retrieved from http://medium.com/personal-growth/13-things-you-need-to-give-up-if-you-want-to-be-successful-44b5b9b06a26.

THE AWESOME POWER OF VISUALIZATION

Goal Setting. *Energizing Goals*. Retrieved from www.learnsellingonline.com/Preview/GoalSetting/07-EnergizingGoals.html.

Hardy, B. P. (2017, July 21). If You Don't Believe In Setting Goals, It's Because You Don't Know How To Do It. *Thrive Global*. Retrieved from https://journal.thriveglobal.com/if-you-dont-believe-in-setting-goals-it-s-because-you-don-t-know-how-to-do-it-cdddea181aab.

Kondo, M. (2014). *The Life-Changing Magic of Tidying up: the Japanese Art of Decluttering and Organizing* (1st ed.). Berkeley: Ten Speed Press.

Murphy, M. (2015, January 20). Passion Is The Missing Ingredient In Goal-Setting. *Forbes Magazine*. Retrieved from www.forbes.com/sites/markmurphy/2015/01/16/passion-is-the-missing-ingredient-in-goal-setting/.

St. George-Godfrey, E. (2014, January 9). Goal Setting, Goal Achievement and the Influence of Emotions. *Kaizen Biz*. Retrieved from http://kaizenbiz.com/goal-setting-goal-achievement-and-the-influence-of-emotions/.

EXAMPLE VISUALIZATION

Irving, M. 'Chili.' (2016). The Energy Rocket. *The Energy Rocket*. Retrieved from www.theenergyrocket.com/. [This is her website, however, she inspired me with her visualization while in Fiji for a Tony Robbins Life Mastery Event in March 2016.]

PART 3: TRANSFORM

Health Canada. (2016, June 9). Food Irradiation. *Canada.ca*. Retrieved from www.canada.ca/en/health-canada/services/food-nutrition/food-safety/food-irradiation.html.

About the Author

Agathe Regina Holowatinc, MLIS, INHC, is a passionate advocate of real food, holistic approaches to health and communicating big ideas in a simple way. She believes that vibrant health is our birthright and that achieving optimal health is the best springboard for achieving all of our biggest dreams. Agathe holds a Bachelor of Arts degree with a Major in Communication from Simon Fraser University and an ALA accredited Master of Library and Information Studies degree from the University of British Columbia. She is also a graduate of the Institute of Integrative Nutrition® in New York and is trained in modern health coaching, eastern and western nutrition philosophies, and relating the impact of dietary and lifestyle changes on optimal health to others. Agathe loves to cook and has spent 20+ years thinking about how she can deliver food that will actually benefit those who eat it -- That will actually FUEL their body. This is her first book.

www.ingramcontent.com/pod-product-compliance
Lightning Source LLC
Chambersburg PA
CBHW051558030426
42334CB00031B/3255